Regulation of the Healthcare Professions

Regulation of the Healthcare Professions

TIMOTHY S. JOST

Health Administration Press
Chicago, IL

01 00 99 98 97   5 4 3 2 1

Library of Congress Cataloging-in-Publication Data

Regulation of the healthcare professions / edited by Timothy S. Jost.
   p.   cm.
   Includes bibliographical references.
   ISBN 1-56793-058-1
   1. Medical personnel—Licenses—United States.   2. Medical personnel—Legal status, laws, etc.—United States.   I. Jost, Timothy S.
   RA399.A3R44 1997
   362.1'0973—dc21   97-2634
                                                                    CIP

The paper used in this publication meets the minimum requirements of American National Standards for Information Sciences—Permanence of Paper for Printed Library Materials, ANSI Z39.48–1984. ∞ ™

Health Administration Press
A division of the Foundation
   of the American College of
   Healthcare Executives
One North Franklin
Suite 1700
Chicago, IL 60606
312/424–2800

CONTENTS

FOREWORD

Richard D. Lamm

CHANGE IS seldom linear. Institutions like nature seem to be subject to what scientists call "punctuated equilibrium" where the status quo is the norm "punctuated" by periods of massive change. Healthcare delivery has gone through a similar process with decades of little or no change in healthcare institutions giving way to today's massive changes. More change has taken place in the organization, funding, and delivery of healthcare in the last four years than in the previous forty. An old world of fee-for-service medicine is dying and a new world of integrated delivery systems and managed care is being born.

When paradigms shift, virtually everything within that paradigm shifts. A society does not go through as massive a movement into this new world of healthcare as the United States has, without it affecting virtually everything within that system. We are in the process of rethinking many of our most basic organizational, regulatory, and ethical institutions. Few elements of the old system will remain unchanged.

How do we reform and modernize all the interrelated parts of the healthcare delivery system? One of the challenges of change is to avoid keeping old institutions intact after change has made them obsolete. Change requires us to focus on substance not form. How do we reform our existing institutions to correspond to the substance of what *is* taking place rather than the form of what *was*?

As we struggle to rationalize the financing and delivery of healthcare, we too often overlook the healthcare workforce. How we educate, train, and use the United States's 10.5 million healthcare workers has a tremendous effect on the cost, quality, and accessibility of our system. Clearly we must change the nature and role of professional regulation. States, which control the education and regulation of healthcare providers, must craft new and assertive public policies to produce a healthcare workforce that can deliver the promises of a reformed system. Some states are responding, and many have realized that by changing education and training, regulation, and licensure, the healthcare workforce can become the foundation of an efficient, high quality, and more equitable new system.

The regulation of the health professions would require review even if the healthcare system was not awash with change. Critics increasingly question the existing health-profession regulatory system. Professions dominate their licensure boards and yet we give them the authority of government and allow them to self-regulate. Is regulation protecting the public or the professions? Licensure can bring higher costs, reduce access, and limit managerial flexibility. Statutes can stymie the optimal use of nurses, physician assistants, and some other providers. State regulatory processes can inhibit the effective deployment of personnel. There are a myriad of old world policies in need of change.

In my experience, regulation has too often served the profession first and the public second or not at all. It has enforced orthodoxy and slowed innovation more often than protecting the public. I seriously question whether, in many areas of regulation, benefits have exceeded costs.

I can't imagine the hours I have spent listening intently to the differences between the ophthalmologist and the optometrists, or the hundreds of hours listening to the turf battles between the various branches of medicine or nursing. Looking back on it, few of these arguments had anything to do with competency or public safety. It was monopoly and money not safety and skills that were usually at stake. Regulation has too often ignored the impaired professional and focused on the endangered income flows; it has been better at continuing the financial exploitation of the profession than in protecting patients from sexual exploitation.

There is a need for creative regulation, perhaps a greater need today than ever. Some professionals will continue to become impaired, obsolete, incompetent, and abuse trust. We shall have to tailor the regulatory system to fit the new realities of healthcare. But we must go back and ask ourselves what we want out of our regulation and how do we resist temptations to misuse regulation.

That is the great contribution of this book. It examines in-depth how the nature and role of regulation has changed. It suggests we need less regulation in some areas and more in others. It analyzes the variety of quality control checks available today that were previously unavailable and shows how this gives the consumer a variety of tools like report cards, HEDIS data, outcomes data, and so on, which directly relate to how we restructure the regulation of the health professions. It examines the promise and dangers of institutional licensure.

Efficient health delivery must allow us to use the appropriate worker for a variety of skills without over intrusive regulation. We have many hospitals in the United States with more job categories than they have beds. A large number of new professions and skills have been created for billing purposes under prospective payment that will have to be rethought. We have to improve our methods of preventing the entrance of incompetent and inadequately professionals trained into healthcare professions, and we have to completely reengineer our system of assurance of continued profession competence after licensure.

The reexamination of the role of regulation in the health professions should not be looked at like a chore—it is an opportunity. We have better safety for the public, with less regulation and less cost to the consumer and less hassle to the profession—if we do this right.

PREFACE

THE DESIRE to create this book grew out of my experience as a consumer member of the State Medical Board of Ohio during the years 1987 to 1992. I was deeply impressed through this experience with the rapid and profound changes that the healthcare professions are currently undergoing and with the need for professional regulatory agencies to respond to these changes. I was also struck, however, with the paucity of accessible literature discussing the ever-more-pressing legal issues and ever-more-challenging technical problems facing the licensure boards and other bodies that regulate the professions. There has been a great deal written on the sociology and economics of the professions and of regulation in recent years, much less written on the practical problems encountered by professional regulators. This book is an attempt to fill that gap.

The subject of professional regulation is immense, and no book of this size can attempt all. In an effort to make the task manageable, this book focuses on professional licensure and pays less attention to the educational institutions that train professionals and form their values, the educational accreditation agencies that oversee these schools, the specialty certification and registration boards that regulate much of specialty practice, and the managed care and hospital certification programs that perhaps currently have the greatest regulatory effect on professional practice.

The book also, perhaps unfortunately, focuses primarily on regulation as it affects a small subset of the many licensed professions that provide healthcare, that is, on physicians, and to a lesser degree nurses, dentists, and pharmacists. The book takes this focus for several reasons. First, most of the court decisions with which the lawyers who write this book concern themselves deal with these professions. Second, the boards that regulate these professions tend to have the most resources and the most sophisticated regulatory programs. Third, professionals in these professions tend more often than others to be in independent practice, not subject to oversight by employers or other institutions, and thus regulatory oversight of these professions is arguably more necessary. It is not our intent, however, to denigrate the importance of occupational therapists, physical therapists, clinical dietitians and nutritionists, clinical laboratorians, health information managers, or other professionals, who deliver much of the healthcare received by Americans. We believe, moreover, that most of what we have to say in this book pertains to these professions as well.

I would like to thank those who supported me in editing this book. First an exceptional group of colleagues wrote the chapters of this book, on time and within their allotted page limits. Second, I would like to thank my former colleagues with the State Medical Board of Ohio, from whom I learned a great deal, especially Ray Bumgarner, the executive director, and Henry Cramblett, an exceptionally professional physician. Finally, I would like to thank those who supported me in this effort, especially my dean, Gregory Williams; Dr. Ronald St. Pierre of the Ohio State University College of Medicine; Professor Dr. Erwin Deutsch of the Universität Göttingen, Germany, in whose Lehrstuhl I worked as I finished this book; my research assistants, Toby Williams and Tracy Kozicki, my secretary Carol Peirano; and my wife, Ruth, and children, Jacob, Micah, and David.

Timothy Jost
Göttingen, Germany 1997

INTRODUCTION—REGULATION OF THE HEALTHCARE PROFESSIONS

Timothy S. Jost

A LITTLE more than a century ago, the United States Supreme Court considered the appeal of a medical practitioner named Frank M. Dent.[1] Dent, a graduate of the American Medical Eclectic College of Cincinnati, Ohio, who had practiced in West Virginia for six years, was refused a license to practice medicine by the West Virginia State Board of Health. The board had determined that Dent was not the graduate of "a reputable school." Dent was subsequently convicted of the unlicensed practice of medicine. Dent, appealing this conviction, argued that, having established a successful medical practice, he had a property interest that the state could not take from him. He attacked the very idea of professional licensure.

Mr. Justice Field, writing for the unanimous Supreme Court, rejected Dent's claim. Justice Field took note of the arcane and complex body of knowledge that physicians must master, and then asserted:

> Every one may have opportunity to consult [the physician], but comparatively few can judge of the qualifications of learning and skill which he possesses. Reliance must be placed upon the assurance given by his license, issued by an authority competent to judge in that respect, that he possesses the requisite qualifications.[2]

In this passage the Supreme Court articulated, at the dawn of modern professional regulation in the United States, both a justification for government regulation of the professions and an understanding of its purpose. The justification was market failure: consumers do not have the information needed to evaluate the competence of medical professionals and are not able to understand such information as is available to them. The Court endorsed the belief that consumers do not have the expertise needed to identify competent medical practitioners. Regulatory intervention is thus necessary to protect them. Based on this belief, the Court defined the purpose of licensure: confirming that professionals "possessed the requisite qualifications" to practice their profession.[3] Licensure, the Supreme Court assured us, was to ensure competence.

Professional regulation was not altogether a recent innovation when Dr. Dent brought West Virginia before the Supreme Court in the late nineteenth century. Professional licensure laws existed in the Holy Roman Empire in the thirteenth century, and the College of Physicians and Surgeons was given authority over medical licensure in England in the sixteenth century.[4] Licensure grew up in the context of the guild system in Europe, with the intimate involvement of the Church and of the universities. Professional regulation was present in some of the American colonies in the seventeenth century, and physician licensure laws became common by the end of the eighteenth.[5] These laws generally vested licensure authority in the medical societies.[6] Despite this early presence, however, professional licensure had been generally abandoned in the United States during the middle of the nineteenth century, a time when medical orthodoxy was weak and populism and egalitarianism were strong.[7] Dent marks the resurgence, therefore, of licensure, though not its birth.

When professional licensure reemerged at the end of the nineteenth century, the battle for its adoption was led by the newly founded American Medical Association (AMA) and its constituent state societies.[8] One concern of those lobbying for licensure was the elimination of competition from unorthodox schools of medicine, such as the Thompsonians or Eclectics.[9] The advocates of licensure were also more broadly concerned with protecting trained medical practitioners, whatever their school of practice, from graduates of substandard medical institutions or from untrained lay healers.[10]

From the beginning, therefore, professional regulation has served not only the public but also professionals and the professions. Though licensure has been directed toward ensuring professional competency, it has also been concerned with maintaining professional identity and orthodoxy, economic power, and social and educational elitism.[11] It has been preoccupied with boundary maintenance—and not just with preserving the borders that separate the laity and the profession, but also with protecting the territory of one profession from that of another.[12] Podiatrists preside over the foot, dentists over the mouth. Physicians rule the entire body, and the uninitiated can have none of it. Licensure laws and boards have defined and enforced ethics—those principles that structure the relationships between professionals and their patients, professionals and the public, and professionals and other professionals. Historically, professional ethics have often been at least as much concerned with preserving professional peace and prerogatives as with protecting patients.[13] Finally, when regulatory boards have undertaken professional discipline, they have focused their efforts on ridding the professions of their failures and embarrassments—rogues, criminals, and charlatans.[14] Competency as such has been less of a concern.

In the second half of the twentieth century, some of these tasks of professional regulation have come under severe attack. Professional regulation has been condemned for contributing to the high cost of professional services, both by creating professional cartels and by blocking the substitution of lower-cost for higher-cost services of equivalent quality.[15] It has been scored for blocking entry into the professions on the part of minorities and the foreign trained, and for hindering the development of alternative approaches to healing.[16] Perhaps most loudly and persistently, it has been criticized as not being competent to ensure competence, and of thus failing in its primary mission.[17]

Despite these charges, professional licensure has endured and indeed flourished. It has survived both the consumer revolution and the deregulation preoccupation of the 1960s, '70s, and '80s. It was, of course, affected by these trends.[18] Licensure boards added consumer members and paid more attention to consumer complaints.[19] Two-thirds of the states adopted sunset laws in the late 1970s, and though relatively few licensure boards were actually terminated, sunset legislation did provide for greater legislative oversight.[20] Other states consolidated boards. Boards were given new disciplinary sanctions and authority, and disciplinary actions based on competency issues increased in frequency.[21] The worst excesses of anticompetitive ethical constraints were eliminated.[22] Foreign-trained physicians gained more equitable treatment (though not necessarily more favorable treatment) with the adoption of a uniform national medical licensure exam (USMLE).[23]

As the twentieth century has progressed, new forms of regulation have also emerged. The federal Peer Review Organization Program has taken on oversight of the quality and necessity of care provided to Medicare patients. Federal regulatory programs are discussed in Chapter 8, written by Mark R. Yessian and Joyce M. Greenleaf. Federal and state fraud and abuse and self-referral laws oversee professional conflicts of interest, as the federal antitrust laws police anticompetitive conduct. The antitrust laws are discussed in Chapter 7, written by Thomas L. Greaney. Public regulation is supplemented as well by an extensive web of private regulation. For some time medical societies have policed the conduct of their members, specialty boards have certified qualified applicants as "board certified," and healthcare institutions have granted staff and clinical privileges. Now managed care plans are also actively engaged in credentialing staff. The focus of this book is on public regulation, but it will touch from time to time on these private credentialing efforts as well, particularly in Chapter 6, by David Orentlicher on the American Medical Association's role in policing ethics and in Chapter 7, by Thomas L. Greaney on antitrust law.

As we near the end of the twentieth century, professional regulation appears on the surface to be as entrenched as ever. Licensure authorities in particular are still firmly in control of entry to their domains, and emerging professions continue to clamor for licensure authority. Yet the handwriting may be on the wall. Professional regulation faces the greatest challenge it has encountered since it surmounted Jacksonian populism a century ago: the emergence of robust healthcare markets.

Even though licensure authority was wrested from the hands of the medical associations a generation or two ago, licensure has remained a creature of professional dominance. In virtually all U.S. jurisdictions, professionals have dominated their own licensure boards, and professional political power dominates licensure policy.[24] Professional power may, however, have reached its limits. The long-heralded proletarianism of the professions seems finally to be under way.[25] In 1994, for the first time in recent history, the real income of physicians ceased increasing; indeed it declined, as more and more physicians forsook their independent practices and became employees.[26] Vigorous markets for healthcare are emerging and driving the organization of healthcare. Healthcare managers, long subservient to healthcare professionals, appear to be gaining the upper hand.

The emergence of sizable healthcare organizations under the control of dominant healthcare managers, whose services are purchased within robust healthcare markets by powerful and knowledgeable health insurers, managed care organizations, and self-insured employers, has momentous implications for healthcare regulation in general, and for licensure in particular. First, if patients can become knowledgeable consumers, if they can be empowered to evaluate comparatively the quality of professional services in competitive markets, is licensure still necessary? If the justification that has served as a bulwark shielding licensure from its foes since Dent crumbles, can licensure long survive? Second, with the advent of robust healthcare markets, the anticompetitive character-istics of licensure that have long vexed its critics become increasingly problematic. Challenges to licensure may intensify at the very time that licensure becomes increasingly difficult to support.

On the other hand, the emergence of healthcare markets may create new roles for professional regulation.[27] Regulatory programs could be-come information generators and processors that would facilitate, rather than frustrate, markets. The regulatory efforts of licensure boards could focus on those areas where markets create rather than solve problems. Significant aspects of professional behavior remain, moreover, that are largely unaffected by markets. Boards retain a vital role in overseeing these areas of professional conduct.

The remainder of this introduction will suggest some of the ways in which emerging markets may change the nature and role of profes-sional regulation. The remainder of the book will explore these topics in greater depth.

Redefining the Role of Professional Regulation in Quality Oversight

In the past, licensure bodies have attempted to ensure the initial compe-tence of professionals by enforcing education and examination require-ments, but largely ignored the problem of ongoing competence.[28] In recent years, boards have acknowledged the need for continual oversight of competence, but have addressed the issue primarily through policing continuing education requirements and through investigating consumer complaints.[29] Neither strategy has been shown to have a significant effect on improving the quality of healthcare.[30]

Though healthcare organizations have to date competed in the mar-ket largely on the basis of cost, competition based on quality is becoming a reality.[31] Employers are increasingly demanding that health plans provide them with Health Employer Data and Information Set (HEDIS) data, which include primitive attempts to provide comparative quality data. The Joint Commission on Accreditation of Healthcare Organizations has begun to publish "report cards" that permit comparative evaluation of the quality of hospitals.[32] In some states and localities, comparative health outcomes data have become available for some conditions and for some providers.[33] Though these data are still primitive, it is hoped that patients and payors may in the not-too-distant future shop for the healthcare provider with the best success rates for dealing with a particular healthcare condition or set of healthcare conditions.

While competition based on quality is still in its early stages, management involvement in quality oversight is advancing rapidly. The continuous quality improvement (CQI) and total quality management (TQM) movements are based on quality improvement and statistical control strategies developed in the industrial setting. The ideas of W. E. Deming, J. M. Juran, W. A. Shewhart, and others had a significant effect on first Japanese, and then American industrial production. Within the past few years, these ideas have begun to be applied widely in healthcare as well.[34]

The quality improvement philosophy defines quality in terms of meeting the needs of "customers," defined broadly to include not only patients but also others who consume the services of the institution, including physicians themselves.[35] It asserts that organizations can be more effective at improving quality, and thus at serving their customers, if they work at improving production systems rather than at looking for "bad apples."[36] One can accomplish more, the philosophy contends, by raising the mean of the performance curve and by narrowing the zone of acceptable variability in performance than by chopping off the tail.[37] Data, and particularly outcomes data, are very important for driving and shaping systems improvement, and a great deal of attention is being given to the identification and refinement of outcome measures both in academic and in practice settings.[38] Not only must systems be monitored continuously, but improvements in systems must also be monitored to ensure that they are in fact effective.[39] Management and staff must be involved at all levels in the process of improvement.[40] The culture of the organization must be molded to emphasize quality.[41] Finally, quality improvement is never finished, there is always room for progress in improving quality.

The rise of market competition and quality improvement management has important implications for licensure. Both market competition and management based on quality improvement, as already noted, create significant demands for the generation, collection, coordination, and dissemination of information. While institutions can be expected to generate their own internal information, the larger job of collecting and disseminating information at the regional, state, and national level will most likely fall to government.[42] This creates significant opportunities for regulatory agencies.[43] Licensure boards are obligated under the federal Health Care Quality Improvement Act to collect and disseminate to healthcare entities information regarding the licensure, credentialing, and malpractice history of physicians.[44] In a few states, they also provide information to the public on these topics.[45] Licensure boards can make a major contribution to facilitating the operation of healthcare markets by participating in this function of creating and processing information.[46]

Second, the emphasis of the private sector on CQI—on polishing apples rather than culling—leaves the government with primary responsibility for identifying and disciplining truly incompetent providers.[47] This task, never a pleasant one, has traditionally fallen to licensure boards. In the past, the performance of licensure boards in this area has often been deficient.[48] But if the task is going to be undertaken (and it must be), it is likely that licensure boards will have to perform it. Their primary competitor for this task, the Medicare Peer Review Organizations, have redefined their mission to focus on CQI, and largely abandoned the culling task (see Chapter 8).

Chapter 2 by Timothy S. Jost and Chapter 9 by Arnold S. Relman directly addresses the future of licensure for quality oversight. Chapter 5 by Eleanor Kinney approaches this topic indirectly, considering the role of licensure agencies in information collection and dissemination.

The End of Parochial Regulation

Licensure has traditionally been parochial in at least two respects. First, licensure in the United States has been a local function. Although there have been proposals for national licensure of professionals for years, they have never gone very far.[49] Professional regulation has always been the province of the states.[50] Second, licensure has been profession specific, with a heavy emphasis on maintaining, and defending, both the boundaries between the professions, and the prerogatives of the more powerful professions.[51]

The market revolution in healthcare has important ramifications for both of these characteristics of licensure. First, it poses serious challenges to traditional scope-of-practice limitations.[52] Healthcare institutions faced with declining operating margins must use their work force as efficiently as possible.[53] They do not have the luxury of employing multiple employees with overlapping skills to perform tasks arbitrarily defined as falling within the domains of different professions. They want to be able to use the least expensive employee who is competent to carry out any particular task.[54] They want to employ professionals who can be used flexibly to carry out a range of tasks.[55] They would like to have the option of training professionals currently associated with the institution to take on additional tasks rather than bring in new staff specially credentialed for these tasks.[56]

Policymakers are responding to these demands. In 1994 alone, 135 state laws were adopted expanding scopes of practice for various practitioners, and the Clinton Health Security Act contained a provision that would have rejected all scope-of-practice limitations that were not competency based.[57] These developments are discussed in Chapter 4, by Linda H. Aiken and William M. Sage.

The local nature of state licensure programs is also increasingly coming in conflict with the demands of a national, indeed an international, market.[58] It is unlikely that state licensure will soon be replaced by a federal licensure program. State licensure provides the opportunity for closer-to-the-ground oversight of professionals, and state agencies are more sensitive to local standards, expectations, and needs.[59] State-level regulation also reflects the continuing strength of professional lobbies and organizations at the state level.

Nevertheless, the federal role in professional regulation is growing. Federal healthcare programs—including Medicare and Medicaid—purchase about one-third of the healthcare consumed in the United States. Through the oversight programs of Medicare and Medicaid, such as the Medicare Peer Review Organization program, and through the regulatory programs that are imposed on the states as a condition of receiving federal healthcare funding, the federal role in healthcare regulation has grown inexorably. The federal Health Care Quality Improvement Act, and the National Practitioner Data Bank it established, have prodded the states toward greater cooperation and coordination.[60] Mark R. Yessian and Joyce M. Greenleaf describe federal regulatory programs in Chapter 8, on federal healthcare regulation efforts. The federal Americans with Disabilities Act, moreover, has imposed federal oversight over state licensure agencies, forcing them to rethink the relevancy of physical and mental limitations for licensure.[61] This act is discussed briefly in Chapter 3 by Sandra H. Johnson.

Coordination among state licensure agencies to achieve national health policy is also becoming increasingly important. The growth of interstate telemedicine, driven largely by the interests of healthcare providers that operate on a regional or national scale, poses a serious challenge to the continuation of state-based licensure.[62] Though it is unlikely that national licensure will soon replace state-by-state licensure, it is likely that the telemedicine issue will force increased coordination among the states and reduce the ability of one state to reject the services of a physician licensed in another.[63]

The National Medical Examination, fully implemented in 1994, is another indicium of an emerging national licensure policy. The increasingly important role of national licensure organizations, such as the Federation of State Medical Boards or National Council of State Boards of Nursing in setting standards for licensure agencies, or of the Council on Licensure, Enforcement, and Regulation and the Citizen Advocacy Center in facilitating communications at the national level between board executives and members will facilitate the national coordination of licensure efforts in a national market. The Pew Health Professions Commission is also making an important contribution in this area.[64]

There is currently a tremendous duplication of effort among licensure and certification agencies, and there are significant opportunities for freeing up resources as sharing of licensure and credentialing data becomes more common and efficient.[65] In the not-too-distant future, greater uniformity of licensure requirements and practices, or perhaps even interstate recognition of state licensure, may permit national medical entities to transfer their healthcare professionals around the country with as little inconvenience as national business corporations now experience in transferring middle-level executives.

There is indeed pressure toward permitting international, and not simply national, mobility. Almost a quarter of the physicians practicing in the United States were trained in other countries, and the number is growing.[66] The General Agreement on Trade in Services (GATS) requires that its signatories, including the United States, ensure that licensure does not impose "unnecessary barriers on trade in services" and specifically further requires that licensure be based on objective criteria and not impose unnecessary burdens on international access to services.[67] The development of the USMLE as a single examination for physicians with foreign as well as domestic training is an important step toward diminishing barriers to the international flow of professional talent.

Regulation of Market Excesses

The maturing of healthcare markets also places new demands on regulatory authorities to address abuses encouraged by markets. One of the most significant issues in this area is conflicts of interest.[68] Interest conflicts are the major focus of the federal bribe and kickback and self-referral laws.[69] Over two-thirds of the states have also adopted laws regulating the financial relationships between healthcare professionals and the entities to which they refer their patients.[70] These laws usually either: (1) forbid professionals from referring patients to entities that they own or from which they receive compensation or (2) require referring professionals to disclose to their patients any ownership interests they may have in an entity to which the patients are referred.[71] Self-referral prohibitions are usually subject to a variety of exceptions for situations in which the financial relationship is unlikely to cause a conflict of interest (e.g., when the professional owns shares in a large, publicly traded corporation) or in which the conflict is practically unavoidable (e.g., when no other providers are available in underserved rural areas).[72] These limitations are often found in licensure statutes, and their enforcement is often the responsibility of licensure agencies.

Self-referral statutes are motivated by the concern that healthcare entrepreneurs might order excessive and unnecessary diagnostic or treatment services for their patients because of their financial interest in the entities providing those services. The incentives created by managed care, on the other hand, tend to encourage the underprovision of care. Professionals or institutions that are financially at risk for the items and services that they provide to their patients are more likely to provide too little rather than too much care.[73] The problem of underprovision can be addressed by licensure boards as a standard-of-care issue when professionals deny services that are clearly necessary, but only the most egregious problems will probably result in disciplinary action.[74] Several states have gone further, specifically adopting statutes regulating managed care plan practices such as limiting access to emergency care.[75] These statutes are usually enforced through insurance departments rather than by licensure agencies. As healthcare markets mature, and the abuses of markets as mediated by professionals become more apparent, licensure boards are likely to be asked to take a more active role in addressing these abuses.[76]

Oversight of Professional-Patient Relationships

Finally, regulatory authorities also have important ongoing responsibilities with respect to aspects of professional behavior that are not primarily controlled by market forces. The patient-professional relationship has always been, and will continue to be, more than just a buyer-seller relationship, and certain professional problems will need to be addressed by extramarket mechanisms.

Licensure boards, for example, have become increasingly sensitive in recent years to their role in protecting patients from sexual exploitation by professionals.[77] Though the power of patients as consumers may be increasing, the professional is inescapably in a position of superior power in the one-on-one relationship with the patient. Too frequently this power has been abused when the professional has used the patient for sexual gratification.[78]

Licensure boards have also become increasingly aware of their responsibility for addressing the problems of impaired professionals.[79] Though in many states, professional societies and institutional impaired-professional committees have taken a leading role in identifying and supervising the recovery of impaired professionals, ultimate responsibility in this area lies with the boards. Licensure boards have become increasingly willing, and able, to address impairment issues.[80]

Licensure boards are also beginning to deal more directly with the problems posed by professionals infected with infectious diseases, in particular human immunodeficiency virus (HIV). In addressing these issues, boards must carefully balance their responsibility to protect patients and the public from infection against their responsibility not to expose professionals unnecessarily to irrational prejudice. They must weigh the patient's right to know against the right of professionals to keep their own medical information confidential.

Boards will also be called upon to police the participation of professionals in end-of-life decison making. When and to what extent is it appropriate for professionals to second-guess the decisions of their patients, or of their patients' families, to terminate treatment? To what extent should professionals assist their patients who decide to terminate life? Should professionals assist the state when it decides to terminate life?[81] All of these are ethical issues that will be presented to regulatory bodies.[82]

Conclusion

Healthcare professions have been with us for a long time. Professional licensure has been with us nearly as long. Indeed, some regard licensure as a defining characteristic of healthcare professions. Insofar as licensure agencies are identified with their traditional roles—policing professional boundaries, protecting professional prerogatives, ousting professionals who embarrass the professions—they seem anachronistic, or at least not terribly relevant to the fast-paced developments the healthcare industry is undergoing.

But if licensure agencies are able to adapt, if they can get out of the way of—or even facilitate—the positive aspects of professional competition; curtail the worst excesses of market-driven professional behavior; and oversee those aspects of professional behavior not subject to market disciplines, then professional regulation has an important, indeed a vital, role to play in our future healthcare system. This book will contribute to discovering and defining this role.

Notes

1. *Dent v. West Virginia*, 129 U.S. 114 (1889).
2. Ibid., 122–23.
3. Ibid., 123.
4. S. J. Gross. 1984. *Of Foxes and Hen Houses: Licensing and the Health Professions.*

Westport, CT: Quorum Books.

5. Ibid. at 52–53; R. C. Derbyshire. 1969. *Medical Discipline and Licensure in the United States*. Baltimore, MD: Johns Hopkins; R. H. Shryock. 1967. *Medical Licensing in America, 1650–1965*. Baltimore, MD: Johns Hopkins Press.

6. J. L. Berlant. 1975. *Profession and Monopoly: A Study of Medicine in the United States and Great Britain*. Berkeley, CA: University of California Press; J. F. Kett. 1968. *The Formation of the American Medical Profession: The Role of Institutions, 1780–1860*. New Haven: Yale University Press.

7. Gross, *Of Foxes and Hen Houses*, 54–55; Derbyshire, *Medical Licensure*, 6.

8. Derbyshire, *Medical Licensure*, 5–7.

9. J. G. Burrow. 1977. *Organized Medicine in the Progressive Era: The Move Toward Monopoly*. Baltimore, MD: Johns Hopkins University Press; Derbyshire, *Medical Licensure*, 7.

10. Burrow, *Organized Medicine*, 58, 61; P. Starr. 1982. *The Social Transformation of American Medicine*. New York: Basic Books; R. Stevens. 1991. *American Medicine and the Public Interest*. New Haven, CT: Yale University Press.

11. See, e.g., Gross, *Of Foxes and Hen Houses*; D. B. Hogan. 1983. "The Effectiveness of Licensing: History, Evidence and Recommendations." *Law and Human Behavior* 7 (2–3): 117; E. Rayack. 1983. "Medical Licensure: Social Costs and Social Benefits." *Law and Human Behavior* 7 (2–3): 147.

12. See, A. Abbot. 1988. *The System of the Professions*. Chicago: University of Chicago Press; B. J. Safriet. 1994. "Impediments to Progress in Health Care Workforce Policy: License and Practice Laws." *Inquiry* 31 (3): 310; L. Prager. 1995. "Licensing Proposals Seek to Overhaul Current System." *American Medical News* 38 (37): 9.

13. J. W. Begun and R. C. Lippincott. 1993. *Strategic Adaptation in the Health Professions: Meeting the Challenges of Change*. San Francisco: Jossey-Bass.

14. L. O. Prager. 1995. "Closer Ties Urged for Societies and Medical Boards." *American Medical News* 38 (18): 3. Improper prescribing (drug pushing) and impairment are among the most common grounds for discipline, while disciplinary actions based on competency are much less common. Office of Inspector General, Department of Health and Human Services. 1990. *State Medical Boards and Medical Discipline*. Boston: Office of Inspector General, 15.

15. C. Cox and S. Foster. 1990. *The Costs and Benefits of Occupational Licensure*. Washington, DC: Federal Trade Commission, Bureau of Economics.

16. S. Dorsey. 1983. "Occupational Licensing and Minorities." *Law and Human Behavior* 7 (2–3): 171; L. Paige. 1994. "Discrimination or Discriminating." *American Medical News* 37 (8): 3.

17. Gross, *Of Foxes and Hen Houses*, 3.

18. B. Shimberg. 1982. *Occupational Licensing: A Public Perspective*. Princeton, NJ: Educational Testing Service.

19. Shimberg, *Occupational Licensing*, 164–68; American Association of Retired Persons. 1987. *Effective Physician Oversight*. Washington, DC: American Association of Retired Persons.

20. Gross, *Of Foxes and Hen Houses*, 111–14; Shimberg, *Occupational Licensing*, 181–82.

21. Office of Inspector General, *State Medical Boards*, 15.

22. See *In re AMA*, 94 F.T.C. 701 (1979), modified & enforced, 638 F.2d 443 (2d Cir.

1980), affirmed mem. by an equally divided Court, 455 U.S. 676 (1982) (striking down AMA advertising and contract practice restrictions).

23. A. J. Cortese. 1992. "New Licensing Test: More Equitable, More Effective." *American Medical News* 35 (23): 33.

24. See Arizona Auditor General. 1995. *The Health Regulatory System.* Phoenix, AZ: Auditor General.

25. See J. B. McKinlay and J. D. Stoeckle. 1988. "Corporatization and the Social Transformation of Doctoring." *International Journal of Health Services* 18 (2): 191; J. B. McKinlay and J. D. Stoeckle. 1985. "Towards the Proletarianization of Physicians." *International Journal of Health Services* 15 (2): 161.

26. M. Mitka. 1996. "Doctor Pay Shrinks for First Time in '94." *American Medical News* 39 (4): 1.

27. See generally, T. Brennen and D. Berwick. 1995. *New Rules: Regulation, Markets, and the Quality of American Health Care.* San Francisco: Jossey-Bass; T. S. Jost. "Oversight of the Quality of Medical Care: Regulation, Management, or the Market?" *Arizona Law Review* 37 (3): 825.

28. D. A. Swankin. 1995. *The Role of Licensing in Assuring the Continuing Competence of Health Care Professionals: A Resource Guide.* Washington, DC: Citizen Advocacy Center; Gross, *Of Foxes and Hen Houses*, 147–51.

29. L. J. Finocchio, C. M. Dower, T. McMahon, C. M. Gragnola, and the Taskforce on Health Care Workforce Regulation. 1995. *Reforming Health Care Workforce Regulation.* San Francisco: Pew Health Professions Commission.

30. T. S. Jost, L. Mulcahy, S. Strasser, and L. A. Sachs. 1993. "Consumers, Complaints, and Professional Discipline: A Look at Medical Licensure Boards." *Health Matrix* 3 (2): 333; Finocchio, *Reforming Health Care Workforce Regulation*, 25–26.

31. D. J. Lipson and J. M. De Sa. 1996. "Impact of Purchasing Strategies on Local Health Care Systems." *Health Affairs* 15 (2): 61, 69–70.

32. See T. S. Jost. 1994. "Confidentiality and Disclosure in Accreditation." *Law and Contemporary Problems* 57 (4): 171.

33. Jost, "Oversight," 837.

34. See e.g., D. M. Berwick, A. B. Godfrey, and J. Roessner. 1990. *Curing Health Care: New Strategies for Quality Improvement.* San Francisco: Jossey-Bass; E. J. Gaucher and R. J. Coffey. 1993. *Total Quality in Healthcare: From Theory to Practice.* San Francisco: Jossey-Bass. One recent survey found that more than two-thirds of the hospitals surveyed were adopting a TQM/CQI program. L. Oberman. 1994. "Quality Quandary: Little Clinical Impact Yet." *American Medical News* 37 (16): 3; P. E. Plsek. 1995. "Techniques for Managing Quality in the Healthcare Setting." *Hospital & Health Services Administration* 40 (1): 50.

35. D. M. Berwick. "Controlling Variation in Health Care: A Consultation from Walter Shewhart." *Medical Care* 29 (1991): 1212, 1214; Gaucher and Coffey, *Total Quality*, 27–28.

36. M. T. Koska. "Discard 'Bad Apple' Theory of Quality Assurance." *Hospitals* 64 (12): 64.

37. S. B. Kritchevsky and B. P. Simmons. "Continuous Quality Improvement: Concepts and Applications for Physician Care." *Journal of the American Medical Association* 266 (13): 1817.

38. See D. M. Berwick et al., *Curing Health Care*, 46–66; K. L. Coltin and D. B. Aronow.

1993. "Quality Assurance and Quality Improvement in the Information Age." In *Putting Research to Work in Quality Improvement and Quality Assurance*, edited by M. L. Grady, J. Bernstein, and S. Robinson. Silver Springs, CO: Agency for Health Care Policy Research; Kritchshevsky and Simmons, "Continuous Quality Improvement."

39. Berwick, *Curing Health Care*, 134–43; Kritchshevsky and Simmons, "Continuous Quality Improvement."

40. See R. F. Casalou. 1991. "Total Quality Management in Health Care." *Hospital & Health Services Administration* 36 (1): 131; Gaucher and Coffey, *Total Quality*, 99–180, 217–45.

41. Berwick et al., *Curing Health Care*, 1214; Gaucher and Coffey, *Total Quality*, 148–80.

42. While much of this information is currently being collected by private credentialing agencies, they are in turn dependent upon government agencies for information. See L. Prager. 1995. "Move to Cut Credentialing Chaos." *American Medical News* 38 (32): 3.

43. Finocchio, *Reforming Health Care Workforce Regulation*, 22–24.

44. 42 U.S.C. §§ 11131-37.

45. Finocchio, *Reforming Health Care Workforce Regulation*, 19–20.

46. See Massachusetts Advisory Committee on Public Disclosure of Physician Information. "Making Informed Choices about Doctors." Report to Secretary of Consumer Affairs and Business Regulation, 1995; Arizona Auditor General. 1995. *Special Study: The Health Regulatory System*. Phoenix, AZ: Auditor General.

47. See T. Brennan and D. Berwick, *New Rules*, 356–59.

48. American Association of Retired Persons. 1985. *Effective Physician Oversight: Prescription for Medical Licensing Board Reform.* Washington, DC: American Association for Retired Persons; Finocchio, *Reforming Health Care Workforce Regulation*, 29–31.

49. J. R. Wynn. 1995. "Endorsement: State vs. National Licensure." *Federation Bulletin* 82 (1): 9; O. L. Zeve. 1993. "Physician Discipline: Considerations for a National Policy." *In the Public Interest* 13: 1.

50. Zeve, "Physician Discipline," 13.

51. Begun and Lippincott, *Strategic Adaptation*, 12, 89–111.

52. See "Pulling for a Piece of the Health Care Market." 1993. *American Medical News* 36 (5): 3.

53. E. Schneller and J. Ott. 1996. "Contemporary Models of Change in the Health Professions." *Hospital & Health Services Administration* 41 (1): 121.

54. Begun and Lippincott, *Strategic Adaptation*, 25.

55. See M. Fottler. 1996. "The Role and Impact of Multiskilled Health Practitioners in the Health Services Industry." *Hospital & Health Services Administration* 41 (1): 55.

56. See Begun and Lippincott, *Strategic Adaptation*, 107.

57. See Finocchio, *Reforming Health Care Workforce Regulation*, 11–13; H.R. 1200, Health Security Act, § 1161 (1993).

58. J. R. Winn. 1995. "Endorsement: State vs. National Licensure." *Federation Bulletin* 82 (1): 9.

59. Ibid.

60. 42 U.S.C. §§ 11101-52.

61. See C. F. Ryland. 1996. "Accommodating the Americans with Disabilities Act in a Licensing and Disciplinary System." *Straight Forward* 7 (Winter): 1.

62. See P. F. Grandade. 1996. "Implementing Telemedicine on a National Basis—A Legal Analysis of the Licensure Issues." *Federation Bulletin* 83 (1): 7; R. del Junco and J. Cordray. 1996. "Telemedicine Prospects and Perils: Weighing the Potentials." *Federation Bulletin* 83 (1): 18; S. S. Huie. 1996. "Facilitating Telemedicine: Reconciling National Access with State Licensing Laws." *Hastings Communications and Entertainment Law Journal* 18: 1.

63. See Granade, "Implementing Telemedicine," 8–14; L. Prager. 1995. "Medical Board Plan Would Speed Telemedicine Licensing." *American Medical News* 38 (40): 4.

64. See Finocchio, *Reforming Health Care Workforce Regulation*.

65. See L. Buckler. 1995. "Medical Licensure in the 21st Century: Are We Ready?" *Federation Bulletin* 82 (4): 203.

66. F. Mullen, R. Politzer, and C. H. Davis. 1995. "Medical Migration and the Physician Workplace: International Medical Graduates and American Medicine." *Journal of the American Medical Association* 273 (19): 1521.

67. Article VI, 4.

68. M. A. Rodwin. 1993. *Medicine, Money, & Morals: Physicians' Conflicts of Interest.* New York: Oxford University Press.

69. 42 U.S.C. §§ 1320b-7(b), 1395nn.

70. J. C. Dechene and K. P. O'Neill. 1996. "'Stark II' and State Self-Referral Restrictions." *Journal of Health and Hospital Law* 29 (2): 65.

71. Dechene and O'Neill, "Stark II," 69–71.

72. Ibid.

73. See P. H. Bucy. 1993. "Health Care Reform and Fraud by Health Care Providers." *Villanova Law Review* 38 (4): 1003.

74. *State of Arizona v. Board of Medical Examiners of the State of Arizona*, No. CV 94-11501 (Ariz. Super Ct. May 18, 1995). (Currently pending before the Arizona Ct. App.)

75. M. Freudenheim. 1996. "HMOs Cope with a Backlash on Cost Cutting." *New York Times* 115 (50,432): 1.

76. See L. O. Prager. 1995. "State Licensing Boards Consider Curbing Financial Incentives." *American Medical News* 38 (39): 1.

77. Ad Hoc Committee on Physician Impairment. 1995 "Report on Sexual Boundary Issues." *Federation Bulletin* 82 (4): 208; R. P. Reaves. 1993. "Sexual Intimacies with Patients: The Regulatory Issue of the Nineties." *Federation Bulletin* 80 (2): 83.

78. G. D. Gabbard and C. Nadelson. 1995. "Professional Boundaries in the Physician-Patient Relationship." *Journal of the American Medical Association* 273 (18): 1445.

79. See, Symposium on Impaired Physician Programs. *Federation Bulletin* 82 (3): 125. 1995.

80. See "Report of the Federation's Ad Hoc Committee on Physician Impairment." *Federation Bulletin* 81 (4): 229. 1994.

81. S. A. Ragon. 1995. "Comment, A Doctor's Dilemma: Resolving the Conflict Between Physician Participation in Executions and the AMA's Code of Medical Ethics." *University of Dayton Law Review* 20 (3): 975.

82. Dr. Kevorkian's license has been suspended by both the Michigan and California boards.

OVERSIGHT OF THE COMPETENCE
OF HEALTHCARE PROFESSIONALS

Timothy S. Jost

MOST PERSONS seek healthcare because they believe (or fear) that something is wrong with them that they want made right. They want information—to know what, if anything, is in fact wrong—and they want effective treatment, if such treatment exists. It is perhaps obvious that these desires are often not fully satisfied. Either the condition cannot be diagnosed with any certainty or it is, in fact, ultimately not treatable.

It is also true, unfortunately, that many persons who seek help from healthcare professionals and institutions not only do not receive help, but are actually harmed by the experience. The Harvard Medical Practice Study, which analyzed the medical records of patients hospitalized in New York hospitals in 1984, found that nearly four percent of the patients suffered an injury during the hospitalization from the medical care they received, and 14 percent of these injuries were fatal.[1] Other studies involving a variety of medical treatment settings have found equivalent or higher rates of error and of iatrogenic injury.[2]

Though the most appropriate definition of the term "quality" in the context of healthcare is much debated, the ultimate test of the quality of healthcare must be outcomes.[3] Encounters with healthcare professionals or institutions that improve the patient's condition to the greatest extent possible, or at least help the patient to understand why the condition cannot be improved, are of good quality. Healthcare that harms the patient is not good quality care.

This chapter considers the role of professional licensure boards in limiting the incidence of poor quality care. It also considers the more modest role that boards may have in improving the quality of care. While recognizing that the initial, and perhaps most important, contribution of licensure boards to quality is the licensure process itself, this chapter discusses that process only in passing. It also does not consider the contribution that other institutions that directly or indirectly regulate professionals, such as Medicare Peer Review Organizations, specialty boards, hospital and managed care credentialing bodies, or professional associations, might make to quality.

Rather, the primary concerns of this chapter are the use of the disciplinary process for addressing professional incompetence and the efforts of the boards to review continuing competence. Most of the chapter focuses on the disciplinary process, through which licensure boards attempt to rehabilitate incompetent practitioners or to remove them from practice, and, perhaps, to encourage competent care. The chapter first describes how the disciplinary process currently functions in competency cases, and then describes how it might be made to function more effectively. After examining the disciplinary process, the chapter briefly considers how boards might review the continuing competence of practitioners on an ongoing basis.

Throughout, the chapter focuses on physician licensure. It takes this approach primarily because far more information and research are available about the disciplinary processes and actions of medical licensure boards than about the processes and actions of other professional licensure boards. Physician discipline (or the lack of it) also receive more attention from the public, the media, and policymakers than does discipline in other professions. Finally, it is arguable that, because physicians practice more independently than do most other healthcare professionals, and because their actions have such significant capacity to cause harm, professional regulation of physicians is worthy of all the attention it receives. In any event, the chapter will focus on physician discipline, but it will try to draw in information concerning the actions of other professional boards where it is available.

The Tasks of Quality Oversight

If, as we posit, quality is first and foremost shown by outcomes, an examination of regulation of the quality of healthcare must begin by considering why healthcare might result in bad outcomes. First, bad outcomes might result because of deficiencies in medical knowledge or because of professionwide failings.[4] Much is not known about the human body and its afflictions. Much of medical care is based on supposition and on unvalidated custom and convention.[5] News accounts regularly report that common medical procedures have been found to be ineffective, or even harmful.[6]

The most appropriate response to pervasive error is probably not regulation, but rather research and education. The programs of the Agency for Health Care Policy and Research that fund outcome studies and the development of practice guidelines exemplify this approach.[7] Only in the area of drugs and devices (where commercial pressure to get new products into the market is intense and the technology for testing products quite well developed) is a comprehensive attempt made to regulate new approaches to treating illnesses and injuries.[8]

Professional licensure boards in particular have only a modest role to play in combating professionwide quality problems. Continuing education requirements—imposed by many state statutes with respect to many healthcare professions—could play a role in disseminating new knowledge and exposing bad practices, though the value of mandatory continuing education is in dispute.[9] Boards may also contribute by forbidding certain practices (such as the use of controlled substances for treatment of weight loss, steroids for enhancing athletic abilities, liquid silicone injections for breast enlargement, or laetrile for the treatment of cancer), where the dangers of the form of treatment are well understood and rapacity on the part of professionals is likely to cloud medical judgment.[10]

Second, suboptimal outcomes may also occur because of errors committed by otherwise competent practitioners or because of faulty systems within otherwise adequate institutions.[11] By definition, 50 percent of medical practice is below average. The best hope for dealing with problems caused by below-average practice by medical professionals is to strive continuously to raise the average standard of practice and to reduce the deviation from the mean at the lower end.[12] This is the job of institutional CQI or TQM programs, which are rapidly becoming standard within the healthcare industry.

CQI and TQM programs, however, exist at the institutional or healthcare-system level. This is appropriate, given the insight on which these programs are based—that quality problems are usually systemic in nature. These programs cannot take the place of licensure boards, which focus on the performance of individual professionals, nor can licensure programs substitute for their systemic focus. The major tasks of licensure programs with respect to institutional quality improvement programs are to assist them in information sharing and to try not to burden them excessively. In their recent book, *New Rules*, Troyen Brennan and Donald Berwick explore the range of contributions that public regulatory agencies and accreditation bodies could make toward supporting these programs and disseminating the innovations that result from them.[13] This ground will not be reexplored here.

Finally, a significant residue of bad outcomes are caused by incompetent professionals. The term "incompetent" is used here to mean professionals who consistently cause harm or fail to provide appropriate care.[14] Incompetence could be attributable to a number of causes: impairment due to physical or mental disability or substance abuse; fundamental lack of adequate intelligence to do the job; superannuation or other failure to keep abreast of developments; chronic carelessness; "burn out" attributable to overwork, personal problems, or other sources; or venality.[15]

No one knows what proportion of professionals are incompetent. Experts in the work of disciplinary boards have estimated that at any one time, 5 to 15 percent of practitioners are incompetent.[16] Though these numbers are not supported by empirical studies, they are plausible. Physician-owned insurance companies, for example, limited the coverage of 2.5 percent of their physicians in one studied year because of competency concerns.[17] Experts in the field estimate the level of physician impairment at 5 to 12 percent.[18] Considering the range of causes that might contribute to incompetence, it is likely that a significant number of professionals are dangerously lacking in competence.

It is unclear exactly how much harm incompetents do, though it is clear that they are a significant menace. Studies of malpractice settlements and judgments show that a high percentage of all payments are attributable to a relatively small number of practitioners,[19] and that, to some extent, past claims are predictive of future claims.[20]

Protecting the public from incompetent practitioners has long been recognized as the primary justification for professional licensure.[21] It can be argued, however, that it is more important today than ever before that boards take on this responsibility. Within the last half-decade, the quality improvement or quality management philosophy, noted above, has swept healthcare. A primary tenet of quality improvement is that efforts should be devoted to improving systems rather than to getting rid of "bad apples." This is very attractive to professionals and institutions, who have never had much enthusiasm for disciplining their peers in any event. But as healthcare institutions, managed care institutions, and now even Medicare Peer Review Organizations, turn away from looking for the bad apples to polishing the good ones, someone must be left to handle the distasteful task of culling. The bad apples still remain.

The culling task, unfortunately, is left to the professional licensure board. The task is twofold: When the incompetent practitioner is salvageable, licensure boards must protect the public from being harmed while the salvage takes place. Alternatively, when an incompetent practitioner cannot be salvaged, the board must take the practitioner out of practice.

The Role of the Professional Licensure Board in Quality Oversight

Ensuring professional competence is the reason, of course, for the educational and examination requirements imposed uniformly by licensure boards. Before a person may be licensed as a physician in the United States, for example, that person must complete an educational program leading to a Medical Doctor or Doctor of Osteopathy degree, complete a period of postgraduate clinical training of from one to three years (depending on the state), pass an examination, and satisfy a screening for "character."[22] Professional education plays a very important role in educating, training, and socializing professionals, and is probably, in the end, the most important determinant of quality. Discussion of the professional education process in the United States, and of the accreditation agencies that regulate it, is, however, beyond the scope of this book.

Policing ongoing competence has historically been the concern of the disciplinary process. Statutes establishing professional regulatory bodies invariably include a list of grounds on which licensure actions may be taken, several of which relate to quality. In physician licensure and discipline statutes, this concern for competence is articulated in several different ways. First, these statutes commonly permit disciplinary actions premised on "incompetence" or "manifest incompetence," sometimes defined in terms such as "continual failure to exercise the skill or diligence or use the methods ordinarily exercised under the same circumstances by a physician in good standing,"[23] "lack of professional competence to practice medicine with a reasonable degree of skill and safety for patients,"[24] or "professional failure to practice medicine in an acceptable manner."[25] They also occasionally stipulate that disciplinary actions based on incompetence can be brought without proof of actual injury.[26] Second, physician licensure statutes also ordinarily permit actions based on "repeated malpractice,"[27] "negligence on more than one occasion,"[28] "repeated negligent acts,"[29] or "a pattern of negligent conduct."[30] Third, disciplinary statutes often permit licensure actions based on a single instance of "gross incompetence,"[31] "gross malpractice,"[32] or "gross negligence."[33] Fourth, a number of physician disciplinary statutes describe specific conduct that is regarded as per se inappropriate, such as administration of laetrile or silicone injections, or the use of steroids for enhancing athletic abilities.[34] Finally, disciplinary statutes invariably permit sanctions for physical or mental impairment, substance abuse, inappropriate prescribing of drugs, or other conditions or behaviors that indicate an inability to practice competently. These grounds usually independently support disciplinary actions without a showing of incompetence.

Despite the obvious intention of legislatures that professional licensure boards deal with incompetence, it is often asserted that professional licensure boards have not been very effective in doing so. The initial licensure process attempts to let only competent practitioners into practice, but does not always succeed in this attempt. Though medical licensure boards, for example, uniformly require physicians to have completed a medical education, they do not themselves independently assess the quality of domestic medical education programs, and have only a very limited ability to assess the quality of foreign medical schools, from which almost one-quarter of the physicians practicing in the United States have graduated.[35] There are serious questions, moreover, as to the validity of the examination process.[36] The objective questions found in licensure exams cannot begin to encompass the range of complexity and the degree of uncertainty encountered in practice.[37] Moreover, the judgment processes that examinations are designed primarily to evaluate—those learned in professional schools—seem to differ from the judgment processes professionals use in practice, as is evidenced by the fact that successful practicing physicians do poorly on licensure examinations.[38] Finally, the fact that a high percentage of examination takers usually pass licensure examinations,[39] and that persons who fail can in most instances retake the examination, underscores the fact that if an incompetent professional is not screened out by the educational process, the examination is unlikely to keep that professional from licensure.

Most criticism has been directed, however, at the disciplinary process. In any given year, only a tiny number of healthcare professionals—a small fraction of the number thought to be, in fact, incompetent—are called to account by professional licensure boards. The popular press routinely reports instances in which professionals guilty of egregious, and often repeated, acts of malpractice escape discipline.[40] Professionals found by licensure boards to have committed acts indicating lack of competence often receive only reprimands or brief probations or suspensions, or escape discipline altogether.[41] The licensure boards are often criticized as bungling and inept, or, worse, as corrupted by a desire to protect peer professionals from discipline and from public exposure.[42] Is this criticism, however, justified? To that question the discussion now turns.

The Professional Disciplinary Process and Competence

In order to evaluate the accuracy of these charges, it is necessary to review the process by which licensure boards deal with the competence of their licensees. For this evaluation, it is useful to separate the disciplinary process into four stages. First, boards must identify professionals with potential competency problems. Second, boards must investigate situations where possible problems have been identified to verify the existence, scope, and severity of the problems. Third, boards must prove that the practitioner is incompetent through procedures that satisfy the requirements of due process. Fourth, and finally, boards must respond to proven incompetence with appropriate sanctions.

Historically, licensure boards relied on complaints to identify problem practitioners. Most complaints received by medical boards are initiated by the consumer public.[43] This is true of boards regulating other professions as well.[44] Some licensure boards have taken steps in recent years to encourage consumer complaints, such as establishing toll-free numbers, accepting anonymous complaints, or protecting the confidentiality of complainants.[45] Increasingly in recent years, however, professional boards have relied also on reports from a variety of sources: courts and law enforcement agencies, federal agencies such as the Medicare Peer Review Organizations or the Department of Health and Human Services, hospitals, or other healthcare entities that revoke professional credentials, reports of malpractice settlements and judgments, or reports of incompetent conduct from other licensees.[46] Federal and state statutes commonly require such reports.

The defining characteristic of the problem-identification process as it exists in most professional licensure boards is the passive role of the board.[47] Most boards are reactive rather than proactive. They simply wait for the complaint to appear, then go out and investigate it.[48] Boards have little control, moreover, over the quality or relevance of the information that they receive. Consumer complaints often involve conduct that is of little interest to the boards.[49] Many of the reports received by the boards are from sources that are compelled to report by statute, and that would rather keep the information private.[50] Some of the information, such as reports of malpractice settlements, is in turn grudgingly received by boards that question its importance or relevance.[51] It is not surprising that the vast majority of complaints and reports do not result in disciplinary action.[52]

Complaints and reports are usually screened initially to verify board jurisdiction.[53] They are often also screened to ensure that the charges are sufficiently important to ground disciplinary action if proven. Initial screening is usually done by board staff, but individual board members or complaint committees do the screening for some boards.[54]

Complaints deemed worthy of investigation are usually assigned to investigators, who collect relevant treatment records, interview complainants and complained-of practitioners, and report back to the board.[55] In some boards, board members themselves take part in the investigation.[56] In states that have a centralized professional licensure agency, its investigative staff pursues the investigation.[57]

Once treatment records and reports are assembled, competency cases are often turned over to professionals for expert review.[58] Some medical boards have employed medical professionals to do this review.[59] More commonly, boards rely on volunteer experts or contract with experts on a case-by-case basis.[60] Alternatively, boards in some situations hold investigatory interviews, in which the professional is summoned before a board committee to explain his or her conduct.[61] Some boards also have authority to order a professional whose competence has been called into question to take a competency examination.[62]

Most complaints are closed without disciplinary action, though sometimes an informal and private oral warning is given to the professional.[63] Validated complaints are referred for prosecution, often based on a preliminary vote of the board.[64] In some states, the complaint must move through a multi-tiered process involving agencies other than the board before disciplinary proceedings can be initiated.[65]

The investigatory process of most boards is largely driven by the initial complaint.[66] The focus of the investigation is not whether the complained-of professional is competent, but rather whether the complaint is valid. Boards usually limit their investigation, at least initially, to the facts alleged in the complaint, and often do not proceed to use the complaint as a springboard for comprehensively reviewing the professional's practice.[67] If a peer expert concludes that in the particular case the complained-of practice was appropriate, or at least not egregiously inappropriate, the complaint is usually closed without further action.

The investigative process is usually limited by chronic shortages in staff and resources.[68] These limitations make it difficult for boards to investigate problem professionals thoroughly and cause long delays in major cases.[69] Resource constraints make it difficult for boards both to investigate complaints and to engage in proactive investigations that go beyond complaints.

If a complaint is validated, the case may move to the disciplinary stage. Usually, at this point, the board summons the resources of the state attorney general's office, which are often only grudgingly made available.[70] Although cases sometimes get to this stage based on a single egregious act of negligence,[71] usually several instances of inappropriate or negligent care will be at issue.[72]

The driving force at this stage is due process. The professional license is clearly property protected by due process; indeed, it is very valuable property.[73] The professional threatened with license revocation will usually resist discipline, ably represented by skilled legal counsel.[74] The disciplinary process usually involves multiple steps—a hearing before a hearing examiner and review by the board, followed often by judicial review at the state trial, appellate, and sometimes supreme court level.[75] In about a third of the states, the board must make its case by clear and convincing evidence.[76] Courts reviewing medical board decisions in some states exhibit little respect for the expertise of the board and a willingness to substitute their own judgment, particularly if the disciplined professionals offer plausible expert testimony in support of their actions.[77]

The disciplinary process is commonly lengthy, tedious, and expensive.[78] Most boards are quite satisfied, therefore, when they can resolve cases through consent agreements, voluntary retirements, or private letters of reprimand.[79] Some states provide for informal dispute resolution processes, intended to promote such resolutions.[80] If the terms of the settlement do not address the underlying competency issues, or the retired doctor simply moves to another state, however, the public is not protected.

If the board determines at the end of the disciplinary process that discipline is appropriate, it must devise an appropriate sanction. Revocation, the traditional sanction, has always been problematic. Because of its seeming all-or-nothing nature, revocation is vigorously resisted and reluctantly applied. Moreover, professionals whose licenses have been revoked can in many states reapply for their licenses after a relatively short hiatus,[81] making the sanction much less effective than it would appear. Boards now have generally available a broad panoply of sanctions beyond revocation, including conditional probation or suspension.[82] Creative boards with adequate resources usually do not face statutory impediments to drafting effective decrees. Boards are often limited in their capacity to supervise probations, however, and often settle for ineffective sanctions in their eagerness to resolve complaints.[83]

In sum, criticisms directed at medical boards are certainly not without substance. There is little reason to believe that boards licensing other professions are doing better than medical boards in addressing problems of competence through the disciplinary process.[84] Ascribing to professional licensure boards the best of goodwill, the approach most of them are taking at this point to deal with competency problems is simply not doing the job. There is, therefore, reason to look for a better approach.

Overseeing Professional Competence Through the Disciplinary Process: An Agenda for Change

How can boards become more effective in addressing the problem of the incompetent professional? This section explores what boards are doing and can do to be more effective in identifying, investigating, disciplining, and sanctioning incompetent professionals.

Identifying Competency Problems

As noted above, most licensure boards rely on public complaints as the primary source for identifying problems. One of the functions of a public licensure board should arguably be to respond to public complaints about healthcare professionals. Public complaints, are not, however, a particularly fruitful source of disciplinary actions. One of the few studies of medical board caseloads found that only 5 of 200 public complaints that the study reviewed resulted in disciplinary action initiated by citation and another two in consent agreements.[85] Investigators personally interviewed 164 of the doctors who were the subjects of the 200 complaints and 80 of the persons who complained (or patients whose care was complained of), spending an average of about 10 hours per case in investigations. The small number of resulting disciplinary actions represented a rather small return on their effort.[86]

Where might boards find more productive sources of information? First, boards might better spend their time tracking what the Federation of State Medical Boards refers to as "markers and indicators."[87] Under the Health Care Quality Improvement Act, boards now receive reports of malpractice settlements and judgments and decredentialing actions taken by "healthcare entities," and can gain access to reports of disciplinary actions taken by medical societies and other medical boards.[88] Federal law also requires the Medicare Peer Review Organizations to report to medical boards exclusion actions that they initiate.[89] Under the laws of some states, boards also receive reports from courts, law enforcement agencies, healthcare providers other than hospitals, and other state agencies.[90]

These referrals and reports tend to be more useful than consumer complaints in identifying problems.[91] The study noted above also looked at 200 nonconsumer reports received by the same board, and found that 24 of these resulted in formal disciplinary actions and 15 in consent agreements.[92] Reports are particularly useful if the board tracks and cross-references them to reveal patterns of questionable conduct. Even more useful would be general requirements of reporting of incidents that might involve substandard care, even if they do not result in disciplinary action, as is required of hospitals in Massachusetts.[93]

Many of these reports are also of limited value, however. A single malpractice settlement or judgment, even a very large one, reveals little about the competence of the doctor against whom it was rendered. Multiple settlements or judgments reveal more, but are more common in some specialties than in others, and may in a particular case simply be the result of an enterprising plaintiff's attorney who was able to identify a cluster of unhappy patients of a particular doctor. Most important, perhaps, malpractice settlements and judgments usually occur long after the incidents that gave rise to them occurred, and are thus of little use for quickly identifying competency problems. Reports of disciplinary actions taken by healthcare entities or medical societies are also of limited value if the records underlying the action are sealed by state peer review privileges.

Some boards are permitted access to the records of the malpractice insurance company when a settlement or judgment is reported. Physician-owned malpractice insurance companies have in fact been considerably more aggressive than medical boards in dealing with insured doctors whose competence is questionable. They either deny coverage or impose restrictions or high deductibles on such doctors.[94] Medical boards that have access to investigations conducted by insurance companies, including the insurers' evaluations of their insureds, have a substantial advantage in seeking quality problems. So do boards that have access to the records and documents of healthcare entity and medical society peer review records.

Ultimately, however, many questionably competent professionals are neither sued for malpractice nor disciplined by peer review bodies. Malpractice suits are normally brought on a contingent fee basis, and thus are only brought if a patient is seriously harmed and a strong case for negligence is presented. Professionals in practices where mistakes do not cause dramatic harm, or who serve loyal patients willing to forgive errors, are seldom sued. Healthcare entities are notoriously reluctant to bring privileging actions, which are contentious and costly, and sometimes "carry along" questionable doctors rather than get rid of them.[95] A small percentage of doctors, moreover, practice without hospital staff privileges, and are thus basically unsupervised.[96]

Further steps need to be taken to identify incompetent practitioners. First, strategies need to be developed to identify professionals who are likely to have competency problems or who are not otherwise subject to oversight.[97] Physicians without hospital staff privileges would be one such group. Physicians without managed care contracts might soon be another. Physicians who are very old or semiretired are at risk for losing touch with practice developments.[98] Physicians who have been out of practice for some time and seek to return to practice might be another such group. Physicians who fall into these categories might be subject to random practice audits (in which a sampling of their records would be subject to peer review) or required to take the Special Purpose Examination (SPEX). Their practices could be visited by undercover standardized patients.[99] The leading example of such programs is the program of the Ontario College of Physicians and Surgeons, which randomly audits the practices of randomly selected physicians and physicians over 70 years of age.[100]

Investigatory proceedings are not bound by the same rigorous requirements of due process to which adjudicatory proceedings are subject.[101] Statutes requiring doctors to submit to investigative mental, physical, or competency examinations when there is reasonable cause to suspect incompetence have been uniformly upheld as constitutional.[102] The law of administrative searches would seem to permit practice audits, especially if done pursuant to a well-thought-out profile of likely problem physicians.[103] The state's interest in ensuring that licensees are competent to practice their profession would seem to be at least as strong as the state's interests that justified the random drug testing of high school athletes in the Supreme Court's recent *Vernonia* decision.[104]

A second strategy would take advantage of information increasingly available through electronic data processing.[105] It has become very common for pharmacies to keep their records on computer. Computerized health insurance claims, including claims to government programs, are also rapidly becoming standard. Computerized medical data are being collected by large health data organizations.[106] Half the states now collect physician-identifiable patient data.[107] Increasingly, managed care organizations are assembling HEDIS data. Widespread use of computerized institutional medical records is not far behind.[108]

Healthcare providers and purchasers already use electronic data extensively to review professional practice. Insurers and managed care plans analyze their claims looking for excessive utilization or fraud.[109] A few are even establishing quality review programs that are claims-data based.[110] It is becoming more common for hospitals to track the practice patterns of their physicians.[111] Some hospitals track clinical data under critical pathways programs.[112] More commonly, hospitals and other healthcare entities focus their data gathering and analysis on specific areas of concern under quality improvement or quality management programs. The Joint Commission is well along in the process of requiring hospitals to collect data on performance indicators.[113] Finally, strategies are being devised for monitoring the quality of ambulatory practice using claims data, for example, to review care received by diabetics.[114]

These data sources could also be used for regulatory purposes. Pharmacy regulators and law enforcement officers are already reviewing pharmacy records to identify abuses involving controlled substances.[115] A number of states also collect data on prescriptions under "triplicate prescription" programs, to monitor illegal prescribing of controlled substances.[116] These data could be scanned, applying a small number of algorithms designed for identifying clearly inappropriate or excessive prescribing practices characteristic of physicians of questionable competence. State Medicaid and worker's compensation claims records could be reviewed electronically to identify questionable patterns of practice. A few states already require insurers to report claims data to central state data banks.[117] Many more states require hospitals to report utilization data.[118] These data could be scanned by computer, looking for clear problems.[119] In the long run, hospitals and managed care providers could be required to analyze computerized medical records, using a set of practice algorithms to identify clear outliers.

Investigating Incompetence

Once a professional is identified whose competence is questionable, investigation should range more widely than simple peer review of a particular problem case.[120] Ideally, the next step would be to build a profile of the professional's practice. With a physician, this profile might be compiled through analysis of computerized claims data reported by insurers or discharge data reported by hospitals. Once such a profile is assembled, investigation can be focused on real problem areas to preserve scarce investigative resources.

If, for example, a particular case, identified as a potential problem through a complaint, mandatory report, or practice audit, seems to involve problems or procedures not normally part of the physician's practice, a small number of the professional's other cases might be reviewed to determine whether the professional is otherwise competent but simply practicing out of the professional's area of competence. Alternatively, if a practice audit reveals that a problem case seems to involve diagnoses or procedures typical of the professional's practice, a broader practice audit or focused clinical exam might be indicated.[121] Observation of the physician's actual clinical practice might also be advisable. The goal of the investigative process should initially be diagnostic. It should attempt to determine whether there is a problem, and, if so, its scope.

The fact that the goal at this point is diagnostic has several ramifications. First, it may not be necessary initially to submit all audited cases to thorough peer review. A quick overview of a sampling of cases might be sufficient to determine whether there seem to be general problems with the professional's practice warranting more thorough review, or whether the practice seems generally to be in order. Even cursory investigations should be documented, however, so that problem cases can be readily relocated if further examination becomes necessary.

Second, it may be easier to ask experts to volunteer assistance for diagnostic practice audits than for prosecutorial testimony. In conducting investigative practice audits, most boards will in fact probably have to rely heavily on volunteer experts. Few licensure boards have the resources to pay experts the going rate for expert opinions. A number of boards have had considerable success, however, in obtaining the assistance of volunteer experts or of medical societies.[122] Maryland's peer review program, for example, uses volunteers from the state medical society to conduct peer reviews of questionable practices,[123] and Ohio's Quality Intervention Program relies on a volunteer panel assembled by the medical board.[124] Florida recruits physicians to evaluate problems by offering continuing medical education (CME) credits.[125] If experts understand that they are being asked to help diagnose a problem practice, and will not be asked to testify in prosecutorial proceedings, volunteers may be even more forthcoming. It is essential, however, that boards who rely on volunteers retain control over the investigatory process, and not delegate this control to professional societies that are not accountable to the public.

Third, the primary focus of the investigation at this diagnostic stage should be to help the professional understand areas where additional education and training are necessary.[126] If only minor problems are discovered, remedial measures short of discipline might be appropriate. Though some boards have abused secret consent agreements and letters of caution, the high costs imposed by full due process proceedings indicate a triage process, in which problems that are readily remediable are handled through informal processes that are closely monitored to ensure future compliance.

Once a problem has been confirmed, a next step could be requiring the professional to submit to a competency examination.[127] This could be a general competency examination, like the SPEX, or a clinical competency examination focused on the specific problem at issue. Such examinations could involve standardized patients, computer simulations, or any one of a number of creative strategies devised for testing competence.[128] Ontario's Physician Review Program has already developed and had positive experience with such an evaluation examination.[129] A battery of such tests for addressing a range of common problems could be developed nationally by national licensure federations. Comprehensive assessment centers might also be used.[130] A number of boards currently have investigative conferences, at which the suspected problem professional is required to appear for a meeting.[131] A focused competency examination would demand little more time from the problem professional and could be much more fruitful in pinpointing a particular problem. A licensure statute could be written to provide that, if the professional failed to pass the competency examination (or perhaps a series of competency examinations), he or she could be subject to discipline on this basis alone.

Disciplining Incompetence

If practice audits and competency examinations reveal a problem not readily subject to monitored educational remediation, the case should move to the disciplinary stage. If a statute were written to permit discipline simply on the basis of failure (or repeated failure) of competency examinations, the disciplinary hearing could be relatively straightforward.[132] If failure of a competency examination is not statutory grounds for discipline, however, incompetence will have to be documented thoroughly.[133]

By this point in the process, however, the areas and cases in which the professional experienced difficulty should be clearly identified. A small but significant number of the most egregious of these cases could be assembled and subjected to thoroughgoing expert review. The testimony provided by such experts would document thoroughly the extent and seriousness of the problem for the education of the hearing officer or board, and ultimately the reviewing court, that ruled on the case.[134] Once so educated, the hearing officer or board would be in a position to craft an appropriate sanction to fit the case.

A full panoply of sanctions ought to be available. First, revocation must be available as a viable option. The first duty of a licensure board is to protect the public, not to protect its licensees. If it appears that a licensee is not salvageable, either because of serious character faults or because of deficiencies of education or skill that are not readily subject to remediation, the license must be withdrawn. Suspension should also be available, but as a remedial rather than a punitive sanction. A professional who has been out of practice for six months while suspended is almost certainly less competent upon returning to practice, unless he or she has pursued remedial education during the interim period. Indefinite suspension, during which a professional must pursue an active and intensive program of focused remedial education, might often be the most appropriate sanction for addressing competency problems.[135]

In many instances, a period of supervised probation will be the most appropriate sanction.[136] It should be accompanied by a focused program of continuing education and active monitoring or supervision.[137] As managed care and integrated delivery systems become increasingly dominant, it will be very important for boards to secure the cooperation of these organizations. These entities could be invaluable allies to boards if they agree to provide closely monitored and supervised practice environments. If, on the other hand, managed care organizations refuse to have anything to do with professionals who are being disciplined, they will place serious barriers in the way of remedial programs. It will be important to provide statutory immunity to those individuals monitoring probation to keep them from being deterred by the potential of liability if the monitored physician injures a patient.[138]

One sanction that is of very limited use for addressing competency problems is the public letter of caution or reprimand. All of us who are parents know that a scolding may make the parent feel better but rarely has much of an effect on the child. A case that is not worthy of a stronger disciplinary action than a warning should be disposed of privately, so that the considerable resources necessary to bring a public action can be devoted to other purposes.

Continuous Competency Evaluation

While licensure boards have fallen far short of the goal of protecting the public from incompetent professionals, they at least express allegiance to this goal. Boards have been far less willing to assume the obligation of ensuring the continued competence of practicing professionals. The primary effort that licensure boards have undertaken in this direction has been to require continuing education. About half of the medical and nursing boards require continuing education.[139] As noted above, however, mandatory continuing education has been much criticized. At best it helps a professional maintain a more current knowledge base, but it does little to ensure that professionals actually practice competently.[140] Studies show little relationship between participation in traditional continuing education and actual quality of care.[141]

An alternative proposal considered in recent years has been that the competence of professionals be periodically reevaluated through reexamination. This proposal has predictably been vigorously opposed by professionals.[142] Taking a professional licensing examination is a grueling experience, and no one wants to do it more than once. There is also reason to question whether written examinations are a very effective means of evaluating the practice of professionals. Such examinations measure only knowledge, not the quality of actual practice, and may not even be very effective in measuring clinical reasoning as it is applied in practice. Finally, many professionals tend to specialize in their practice; thus, an examination of general skills would be both a frustrating experience and unenlightening about most of the professional's actual competence in practice.

Some mechanism for ensuring continued competence is, however, necessary.[143] It is fatuous to believe that, once licensed, a professional remains competent forever. It should be clear, moreover, that the disciplinary system cannot be relied on totally to identify professionals lacking competence or to correct gaps in the competence of otherwise competent professionals. The growing interest on the part of employers and managed care organizations in the quality of healthcare also calls for the development of tools for evaluating continued competence. The National Council on Quality Assurance, which accredits managed care organizations, requires accredited organizations both to credential the professionals who practice within them and to evaluate the quality of the care they provide. These organizations will in turn demand evidence of continued competence on the part of professionals.

Most medical specialty societies, following the lead of the American Academy of Family Practice, now require periodic recredentialing, though most grandfather in specialists who were certified when the recredentialing requirements went into effect.[144] The National Council of State Boards of Nursing has acknowledged the importance of continuing competency evaluation and currently has a task force at work developing a nursing regulatory model for continuing competence.[145] The American Association of Dental Examiners has also adopted a position in favor of continuing competency examination and is developing criteria and mechanisms for implementing this position.[146]

As of this point, there is no single strategy emerging for evaluating quality of care on an ongoing basis. For the time being, however, the following principles should be considered in pursuing competency reevaluation strategies:

1. Competency evaluation should take place on a regular and periodic basis. Specialty boards commonly recredential on a seven-year to ten-year basis.

2. Competency evaluation should look at actual outcomes and processes of care, rather than be limited to evaluation of general knowledge.

3. Competency evaluation should focus on the particular area of practice in which the practitioner is actually engaged and not generally attend to areas of practice the professional does not pursue. Some professions, most notably nursing and dentistry, already license on a specialized basis. Perhaps specialty licensure for physicians, or at least licensure to perform broad subcategories of services, should be reconsidered.[147]

4. For the time being, a variety of mechanisms should be available for evaluating competence.[148] Unless and until one strategy for competency evaluation emerges as clearly superior to others, a menu of options should be made available, including traditional examination, practice audit, computerized skill assessment, evaluation using standardized patients, peer review, practice review, clinical case review, and others.[149] The licensure board should be responsible for ensuring that the mechanisms used meet at least minimal standards of validity and reliability and that they are administered with integrity. Use of a range of mechanisms will also provide the opportunity for continuing research and development in this area.

Agencies supervising competency evaluation should responsibly delegate this task when possible, to avoid wasteful duplication of effort and to take full advantage of the exertions and expertise of others.[150] If practitioners are recredentialed by specialty societies through procedures that are methodologically sound and that are carried out with integrity, this recredentialing should be accepted as adequate evidence of competence. It may also be possible to accept credentialing by managed care organizations as acceptable evidence of continued competence, if credentialing is based on actual review of care rather than simply a paper-shuffling process.[151]

Conclusion

Though ensuring the quality of professional practice has long been regarded as the primary justification for licensure, licensure boards are probably not, in the end, the most important institutions available for ensuring quality. What boards can do is to try to address issues of professional competence. Historically, however, they have not been very successful even in doing this. Emerging technologies show great promise for permitting boards to be more effective both at ensuring ongoing competence and at identifying and dealing with practitioners who are not competent. In today's deregulatory environment, boards can no longer afford to fail to fulfil their responsibilities in this key area. This chapter points the way for boards to move forward toward becoming competent in fulfilling their central responsibility of oversight of professional competence.

Notes

1. Harvard Medical Practice Study. 1990. *Patients, Doctors, and Lawyers: Medical Injury, Malpractice Litigation, and Patient Compensation in New York*. Cambridge, MA: Harvard Medical Practice Study, 6–1.

2. L. L. Leape. 1994. "Error in Medicine." *Journal of the American Medical Association* 272 (23): 1851.

3. The Institute of Medicine's 1990 study, *Medicare: A Strategy for Quality Assurance*, identified over 100 definitions of quality of care from relevant literature. The definition that it proposed is, "quality of care is the degree to which health services for individuals and populations increase the likelihood of desired health outcomes and are consistent with current professional knowledge." Institute of Medicine. 1990. *Medicare: A Strategy for Quality Assurance* vol. 1, at 19. Washington, DC: National Academy Press.

4. S. Gorovitz and A. MacIntyre. 1976. "Toward a Theory of Medical Fallibility." *Journal of Medicine and Philosophy* 1 (1): 51.

5. J. Burnum. 1987. "Medical Practice a la Mode." *New England Journal of Medicine* 317 (19): 1220.

6. Ibid.

7. See C. Marwick. 1993. "Federal Agency Focuses on Outcomes Research." *Journal of the American Medical Association* 270 (2): 164.

8. See D. Eddy. 1982. "Clinical Policies and the Quality of Clinical Practice." *New England Journal of Medicine* 307 (6): 343 (describing the problematic process through which clinical standards are developed in medical practice generally.)

9. J. M. Eisenberg. 1986. *Doctors' Decisions and the Cost of Medical Care*. Ann Arbor, MI: Health Administration Press; D. A. Davis, M. A. Thompson, A. D. Oxman, and R. B. Haynes. 1992. "Evidence for the Effectiveness of CME—A Review of 50 Randomized Control Trials." *Journal of the American Medical Association* 268 (9): 1111.

10. See, e.g., Cal. Bus. & Prof. Code § 2251 (liquid silicone injections); Fla. Stat. Ann. § 459.015(v) (prescribing laetrile); Nev. Rev. Stat. § 630.306(4) (liquid silicone injections).

11. See Leape, "Error in Medicine."

12. M. Berwick. 1989. "Continuous Improvement as an Ideal in Medical Care." *New England Journal of Medicine* 320 (1): 53.

13. T. Brennan and D. M. Berwick. 1995. *New Rules*. San Francisco: Jossey-Bass.

14. See M. M. Rosenthal. 1995. *The Incompetent Doctor, Behind Closed Doors*. Buckingham, United Kingdom: Open University Press.

15. Ibid. See also D. A. Morowitz. 1993. "Identification of Physician Incompetence:

The Ethical Dilemmas." *Humanist* 53 (4): 9.

16. See R. Feinstein. 1985. "The Ethics of Professional Regulation." *New England Journal of Medicine* 312 (12): 801; R. C. Derbyshire. 1983."How Effective is Medical Self-Regulation." *Law & Human Behavior* 7 (2–3): 193, 195. Derbyshire, a former member of the New Mexico Board of Medical Examiners and past president of the Federation of State Medical Boards claims without citation that the lower figure has been affirmed by an official of the then Department of Health, Education, and Welfare and the AMA. R. C. Derbyshire. 1983. "The Incompetent Physician." *Hospital Practice* 18 (11): 30, 31.

17. W. B. Schwartz and D. N. Mendleson. 1989. "The Role of Physician-Owned Insurance Companies in the Detection and Deterrence of Negligence." *Journal of the American Medical Association* 262 (10): 1342. See also A. D. Crowe. 1991. "Medical Liability Insurance Companies: Their Role in Delineating Practice." *Federation Bulletin* 78 (7): 208.

18. C. K. Morrow. 1984. "Doctors Helping Doctors." *Hastings Center Report* 14 (6): 32.

19. See U.S. Office of Technology Assessment. 1988. *The Quality of Medical Care, Information for Consumers*. Washington, DC: U.S. Government Printing Office.

20. R. Bovbjerg and K. Petronis. 1994. "The Relationship Between Physicians' Malpractice Claims History and Later Claims." *Journal of the American Medical Association* 272 (18): 1421; J. E. Rolph, D. Pekelney, and K. McGuigan. 1993."Amending the National Practitioner Data Bank Reporting Requirements: Are Small Claims Predictive of Large Claims." *Inquiry* 30 (4): 441; F. A. Sloan, P. M. Mergenhagen, W. B. Burfield, R. R. Bovbjerg, and M. Hassan. "Medical Malpractice Experience of Physicians, Predictable or Haphazard?" *Journal of the American Medical Association* 262 (23): 3291.

21. See, S. L. Baker. 1984. "Physician Licensure Laws in the United States, 1865–1915." *Journal of the History of Medicine and Allied Science* 39 (23): 173.

22. Office of Inspector General, U.S. Department of Health and Human Service. 1986. *Medical Licensure and Discipline: An Overview*. Boston: Office of Inspector General; American Medical Association Council on Medical Education. 1988. "Report on Medical Licensure." *Journal of the American Medical Association* 259 (13): 1994, 1995.

23. Nev. Rev. Stat. § 630.306.7.

24. C. Gen. Stat. § 90-14(a)(11).

25. Tex. Rev. Civ. Stat. Ann. art. 4495b § 3.08 (18).

26. Minn. Stat. Ann. § 147.091(g).

27. Fla. Stat. Ann. § 459.015 (defined as three or more claims in the preceding five-year period resulting in payments in excess of $10,000 each.).

28. N.Y. Educ. Law. art. 131-A, § 6530(3).

29. Cal. Bus. & Prof. Code § 2234(c).

30. Neb. Rev. Stat. § 71-147(5).

31. Ibid.

32. Tenn. Code Ann. § 63-6-214.

33. N.Y. Educ. Law art. 131-A, § 6530(4).

34. Cal. Bus. & Prof. Code § 2251 (liquid silicone injections); Fla. Stat. Ann.

§ 459.015(v) (prescribing laetrile); Nev. Rev. Stat. § 630.306(4) (liquid silicone injections).

35. As of 1988, only ten licensure boards attempted to maintain lists of approved foreign medical schools. American Medical Association Council on Medical Education. 1995. "Report on Medical Licensure." See also, Office of Inspector General, U.S. Department of Health and Human Services. 1986. *Medical Licensure and Discipline: An Overview.* Boston: Office of Inspector General, i, 5–6, 12; A. Skolnick. 1995. "Government Report Gives Department of Education and Some Offshore Medical Schools Failing Grades." *Journal of the American Medical Association* 273 (15): 1162.

36. See R. Tamblyn. 1994. "Is the Public Being Protected? Prevention of Suboptimal Medical Practice Through Training Programs and Credentialing Examinations." *Evaluation & the Health Professions* 17 (2): 198; M. T. Kane. 1992. "The Assessment of Professional Competence." *Evaluation & the Health Professions* 15 (2): 153; W. C. McGaghie. 1980. "The Evaluation of Competence." *Evaluation & the Health Professions* 3 (3): 289.

37. See M. T. Kane, "Assessment of Professional Competence," 177–80.

38. See G. H. Deckert. 1991. "Will Certifying Examinations Ever Predict Physician Performance." *Federation Bulletin* 78 (12): 355.

39. Ninety-six percent of first-time takers and 77 percent of repeat takers passed the NBME Part III in 1994. National Board of Medical Examiners.1995. *1994 Annual Report.* Philadelphia, PA: National Board of Medical Examiners.

40. See, e.g., J. A. Flanery and D. Henless. 1993. "Doctors Unchecked." *Omaha World-Herald*, Feb. 28—March 1; G. O'Neill. 1994. "Malpractice in Massachusetts." *Boston Sunday Globe*, Oct. 2, 30; S. Miller. 1995. "Two Feet of Mistakes." *Newsweek* 125 (13): 60.

41. Only 26 percent of physicians disciplined by state boards in 1995 had their licenses removed, even temporarily. "13,012 Questionable Doctors." *Public Citizen Health Research Group Health Letter* 12 (4): 3.

42. See, e.g., S. Gross. 1984. *Of Foxes and Hen Houses: Licensing and the Health Professions.* Westport, CT: Quorum Books; 1993. "Keeping Doctors Honest: Most Medical Boards Fail the Test." *Public Citizen's Health Research Group Health Letter* 9 (3): 4–7; M. Crane. 1989. "Why Did It Take So Long to Nail This Crooked Doctor?" *Medical Economics* 66 (March 20): 54.

43. Federation of State Medical Boards. 1994. *Final Report on the Strengths and Weaknesses of State Medical Boards as Reflected in the Self-Assessment Instrument and on Proposed Education Programs Based on SAI Data.* Euless, TX: Federation of State Medical Boards.

44. P. C. Damiano, D. A. Shugars, and J. R. Freed. 1993. "Assessing Quality in Dentistry." *Journal of the American Dental Association* 124 (7): 113, 128.

45. Office of the Inspector General. 1987. *Medical Licensure and Discipline*, 15. American Association of Retired Persons (AARP). 1987. *Effective Physician Oversight.* Washington, DC: AARP.

46. See Federation of State Medical Boards. 1995. *1995–1996 Exchange: Section 3: Licensing Boards, Structure and Disciplinary Functions.* Euless, TX: Federation of State Medical Boards, 38–41 (identifying sources that must report to boards.)

47. Only 15 of the 39 boards that responded to the self-assessment instrument

recently distributed by the Federation of State Medical Boards stated that they had attempted to identify problem physicians proactively. Of these only three boards conducted practice audits and three morbidity/mortality studies. The remaining 14 examined prescribing patterns. "39 State Boards Conduct Self-Examinations." *Action Report, Medical Board of California*, Supplement. April 1995: iii; Federation, "Strengths and Weaknesses," 5.

48. R. J. Kinkel and N. C. Josef. 1991. "Disciplining Doctors: How Medical Boards Are Dealing with Problem Physicians in the Midwest." *Research in Sociology in Health Care* 4: 207, 217.

49. Some boards investigate as few as seven percent of complaints. Federation, *Strengths and Weaknesses*, 6. While over 50 percent of complaints come from consumers, only about one-fifth of disciplinary actions are the result of consumer complaints. Ibid.

50. J. Gray and E. Zicklin. 1992. "Why Bad Doctors Aren't Kicked Out of Medicine." *Medical Economics* 69 (Jan. 20): 126; A. L. Hyams. 1989. "Encouraging Hospital Cooperation with a Board's Traditional Disciplinary Functions." *Federation Bulletin* 76 (10): 301; C. L. Rosenberg. 1984. "Why Doctor-Policing Laws Don't Work." *Medical Economics* (March 5): 84, 86–87.

51. See D. Breaden. 1980. "Research in the Sociology of Health Care." *Federation Bulletin* 79 (2): 68, 71 (acknowledging the weaknesses of these data as indicators of incompetence).

52. Federation, "Strengths and Weaknesses." Only about eight percent of complaints result in discipline. Ibid., 6.

53. About 29 percent of complaints are dismissed or referred, "39 State Boards," iii.

54. See R. Cohen and M. Rose. 1993. *Allocation of Decision-Making Authority Between Board Members and Staff*. Washington, DC: Citizens Advocacy Center, 4; Illinois. *Rules for the Administration of the Medical Practice Act of 1987*, § 1285.215.

55. See Wisconsin Medical Examining Board. 1994. *Wisconsin Statutes and Administrative Code, Relating to the Practice of Medicine*. Madison, WI: Medical Examining Board, 137; "When a Complaint Is Received on a Physician." *Nevada State Board of Medical Examiners, Newsletter* 8 (Oct. 1992): 3.

56. Wyoming Board of Medicine. *Rules and Regulations for Physicians and Physicians Assistants* ch. 4, § 4(e).

57. AARP, *Effective Physician Oversight*, 24.

58. See "Board Adopts Major Overhaul . . . Improvements in Use of Experts, Consultants." *Action Report, Medical Board of California* (Oct. 1994): 4.

59. See W. I. Weiss. 1994. "The Evolution of a Medical Director: Experiences of the First Medical Director of the New Jersey State Board of Medical Examiners." *Federation Bulletin* 81 (1): 19, describing the functioning of one board's medical director.

60. Md. Admin. Code tit. § 14-404(a)B; Florida Agency for Health Care Administration. 1995. "1994 Annual Disciplinary Report," 4–6.

61. See N.C. Admin. Code tit. 21, § 32N.0005; L. P. Newton and N. E. Stratas. 1994. "Review of Informal Interviews and Disciplinary Actions by the North Carolina Board of Medical Examiners, 1988–1991." *Federation Bulletin* 81 (1): 23.

62. Federation, *Exchange*, 66–67. See *Smith v. Board of Medical Quality Assurance*, 248

Cal. Rptr. 704 (1988) (upholding constitutionality of required assessment). An examination specifically developed and commonly used for this purpose is the Special Purpose Examination or SPEX. See J. H. Morton. 1993. "The Current Status of Spex." *Federation Bulletin* 80 (4): 257.

63. About 4.5 percent of complaints lead to prehearing stipulations or consent orders, only 2.1 percent go to formal hearings. Overall, about 3.5 percent of complaints result in disciplinary actions, "39 State Boards," iii.

64. Cohen and Rose, "Allocation of Decision-Making Authority," 5. See *Lyness v. Commonwealth State Bd. of Medicine*, 605 A.2d 1204 (Pa. 1992) (finding the boards vote to initiate proceedings was prosecutorial in nature, and thus its subsequent adjudication of guilt violated due process because of the combination of functions).

65. Office of Inspector General, Department of Health and Human Services. 1990. *State Medical Boards and Medical Discipline*. Boston: Office of Inspector General.

66. See, e.g., J. H. Morton. 1991. "Physician Discipline—New York Style." *Federation Bulletin* 78 (5): 143 (describing such a process).

67. Some state statutes, indeed, limit the ability of boards to review the records of patients not involved in the incident being investigated. Office of Inspector General, *State Medical Boards*, 9.

68. Ibid., 7.

69. L. J. Finocchio, C. M. Dower, T. McMahon, C. M. Gragnola, and the Taskforce on Health Care Workforce Regulation. 1995. *Reforming Health Care Workforce Regulation*. San Francisco: Pew Health Professions Commission; E. Graddy and M. B. Nichol. 1990. "Structural Reforms and Licensing Board Performance." *American Politics Quarterly* 18 (3): 376.

70. Office of Inspector General, *State Medical Boards*, 8; Federation, *Exchange*, 18 (about three-quarters of state boards represented by attorney general).

71. See *Tomlinson v. Washington Dental Disciplinary Board*, 754 P.2d 109 (Washington 1988); *Rosi v. State Medical Board*, 665 P.2d 28 (Alaska 1983); *Yellen v. Board of Medical Quality Assurance*, 220 Cal. Rptr. 426 (Cal. App. 1985).

72. *Loffredo v. Sobol*, 600 N.Y.S.2d 507 (N.Y. App. Div. 1993) (gynecologist found to have mistreated nine patients); In re Schramm, 414 N.W.2d 31 (S.D. 1987) (dentist found negligent in 13 cases); *Foltman v. Board of Regents*, 469 N.Y.S.2d 201 (1983) (nurse found to have practiced negligently in six instances).

73. See *Greene v. McElroy*, 370 U.S. 474, 492 (1959); *Beuchamp v. De Abadia*, 779 F.2d 773, 774 (1st Cir. 1985); *Keney v. Debyshire*, 718 F.2d 352, 354 (10th Cir. 1983).

74. Rosenberg, "Doctor-Policing Laws," 89.

75. Gray and Zicklin, "Bad Doctors." See Federation, *Exchange*, 50–51, identifying role of boards and hearing officers in disciplinary actions.

76. Federation, *Exchange*, 72; Inspector General, *State Medical Boards*, 9–10.

77. See, e.g., In re Williams, 573 N.E.2d 638 (1991); *Sizemore v. State Board of Dental Examiners*, 747 S.W.2d 389 (1987). R. C. Derbyshire. 1993. "Obstacles to Enforcement of Discipline." *Hospital Practice* 19 (10): 251.

78. R. Kusserow, E. Handley, and M. Yessian. 1987. "An Overview of State Medical Discipline." *Journal of the American Medical Association* 257 (6): 820. The average board needs 27 weeks to close or dismiss a complaint, 37 weeks to negotiate a stipulation or consent agreement, 47 weeks to complete a hearing. "39 Medical

Boards," iii. Only 69 percent of cases are closed within a year. Federation, *Strengths and Weaknesses*, 6.

79. D. Swankin and S. Willette. 1993. *Should the Public Have a Right to Comment on Proposed Licensing Board Consent Orders*. Washington, DC: Citizens Advocacy Center. Consent agreements are more common than disciplinary actions, and are becoming more common. Inspector General, *State Medical Boards*, 14. The vast majority of informal actions are confidential. "39 State Boards," iii.

80. Tex. Rev. Civ. Stat. Ann. art. 4495b § 4.025(a); Federation, *Exchange*, 52–53.

81. Federation *Exchange*, 67. See Texas Rev. Civ. Stat. Ann. art. 4495b, § 4.10 (licensee whose license is revoked can reapply after one year); Wyoming Stat. § 33-26-406 (revokee can reapply after six months).

82. Federation *Exchange*, 54–55; See, e.g., Conn. Gen. Stat. Ann. ch. 368a § 19a-17; Hawaii Rev. Stat. § 453-8.2; Minn Stat. Ann. § 147.141.

83. I. VanTuinen. 1991. *9479 Questionable Doctors Disciplined by States or the Federal Government*. Washington, DC: Public Citizen's Health Research Group. Only 40 percent keep records on, monitor, and track all physicians in rehabilitation from impairment. Federation, *Strengths and Weaknesses*, 8.

84. See Damiano et al., "Assessing Quality in Dentistry."

85. T. S. Jost, L. Mulcahy, S. Strasser, and L. Sachs. 1993. "Consumers, Complaints, and Professional Discipline: A Look at Medical Licensure Boards." *Health Matrix* 3 (2): 309, 330.

86. Ibid., 329.

87. See Breaden, "Concentrating," 69; B. L. Galusha. 1989. "Perspectives in Medical Discipline, Concentrating on the Problem Physician." *Federation Bulletin* 76 (1): 14, 19–20.

88. 42 U.S.C. §§ 11131, 11132.

89. 42 U.S.C. § 1320c-9(b)(1)(D).

90. Federation, *Exchange*, 38–39.

91. This is not to say that consumer complaints should be ignored. Licensure boards are public agencies and must be responsive to the public. But many consumer complaints could be better handled though other approaches, such as mediation. See Finocchio, *Reforming Health Care Workforce Regulation*, 33.

92. Jost et al., "Consumer Complaints," 331.

93. These include unplanned fractures, postsurgical abscesses, or unplanned transfers to a hospital precipitated by an invasive procedure performed in a physician's office. Office of Inspector General, Department of Health and Human Services. 1991. *Quality Assurance Activities of Medical Licensure Authorities in the United States and Canada*. Boston: Office of Inspector General. 4, A-2–A-3; L. O. Prager. 1995. "What Oversight May Be Overlooking." *American Medical News* 38 (June 5): 1.

94. See W. B. Schwartz and D. N. Mendelson. "The Role of Physician-Owned Insurance Companies" and W. B. Schwartz and D. N. Mendelson. 1989. "Physicians Who Have Lost Their Malpractice Insurance." *Journal of the American Medical Association* 262 (10): 1335.

95. See M. M. Rosenthal. 1995. *The Incompetent Doctor*. Buckingham, United Kingdom: Open University Press, 58–61 (describing this phenomena in England.)

Historically, hospitals were more likely to get a doctor to leave quietly, and thus pass the problem on to others. This is more difficult under the Health Care Quality Improvement Act, which requires reporting of resignations taken under the threat of disciplinary action, but the practice still probably takes place.

96. Though most doctors have staff privileges, in some contexts the number of doctors without privileges can be quite high. A recent study of high-volume Medicaid providers in New York City, for example, found that only 49 percent had hospital admitting privileges. G. Fairbrother, K. A. DuMont, S. Friedman, and K. S. Lobach. 1995. "New York City Physicians Serving High Volumes of Medicaid Children: Who Are They and How Do They Practice?" *Inquiry* 32 (3): 345.

97. See C. Rettie. 1991. "Evaluating the 'At Risk' Physician," *Federation Bulletin* 78 (12): 365.

98. See D. A. Davis, G. R. Norman, A. Poinvich, E. Lindsey, M. S. Ragbreev, and D. Rath. 1990. "Attempting to Ensure Physician Competency." *Journal of the American Medical Association* 263 (15): 2041.

99. The use of undercover agents for identifying doctors guilty of misprescribing controlled substances is not uncommon for boards. See O. White. 1994. "Problem Doctors Aren't Ignored Here." *Medical Economics* 71 (Feb. 21): 99.

100. Inspector General, *Quality Assurance Activities*, B-4–B-5.

101. *Hannah v. Larche*, 363 U.S. 420, 442 (1960).

102. *Humenansky v. Minnesota Board of Medical Examiners*, 525 N.W.2d 559 (Minn. App. 1994); *Smith v. Board of Medical Quality Assurance*, 248 Cal. Rptr. 704 (Cal. App. 1988); *Alexander D. v. State Board of Dental Examiners*, 282 Cal. 3d 201 (Cal. App. 1991); *Gilmore v. Composite State Board of Medical Examiners*, 254 S.E.2d 365 (Ga. 1979).

103. *Marcowitz v. Dept. of Public Health*, 435 N.E.2d 1291, 53 A.L.R.4th 1157 (1982); *Costantini v. Medical Board of Calif*, 34 F.3d 1071 (9th Cali. 1994) (unpublished). See *New York v. Burger*, 482 U.S. 691 (1987) (authorizing warrantless searches in closely regulated industries where there is a substantial government interest in the subject of the inspection, the inspections are necessary to further the regulatory scheme, the owner is aware that his business will be subject to periodic searches, and searches are carefully limited in time, place, and scope.)

104. 115 S.Ct. 2386 (1995).

105. See M. A. Friedman. 1995. "Issues in Measuring and Improving Health Care Quality." *Health Care Financing Review* 16 (4): 1, 9–11.

106. Institute of Medicine. 1994. *Health Data in the Information Age*. Washington, DC: National Academy Press, 29–33.

107. See Note. 1992. "Provider-Specific Quality-of-Care Data: A Proposal for Limited Mandatory Disclosure." *Brooklyn Law Review* 58 (1): 85, 97–98.

108. See R. I. Field. 1994. "Overview: Computerized Medical Records Create New Legal and Business Confidentiality Problems." *Health Span* 11 (8): 3.

109. G. Borzo. 1994. "Smart-Bombing Fraud: Insurers Turn to Powerful New Computer Tools to Spot 'Aberrant' Claims." *American Medical News* (Oct. 10): 3.

110. S. Leatherman, E. Peterson, L. Heinen, and L. Qualm. 1991. "Quality Screening and Management Using Claims Data in a Managed Care Setting." *Quality Review Bulletin* 17 (11): 349–56.

111. See F. Jones. 1994. "Practice Pattern Analysis: A Tool for Continuous Improvement of Patient Care Quality." *Physician Executive* 20 (4): 37.

112. M. Ruffin. 1995. "Physician Profiling: Trends and Implications." *Physician Executive* 21 (11): 34.

113. A. Skolnick. 1993. "Joint Commission Will Collect, Publicize Outcomes." *Journal of the American Medical Association* 270 (2): 165.

114. See J. Weiner, S. Parenete, D. Garnick, J. Fowles, A. Lawthers, and R. H. Palmer. 1995. "Variation in Office-Based Quality, A Claims-Based Profile of Care Provided to Medicare Patients with Diabetes." *Journal of the American Medical Association* 273 (19): 1503.

115. Finocchio, *Reforming Health Care*, 33; Pharmacy Law Digest, PI-9–PI-11. Some medical boards randomly audit pharmacy records, Office of Inspector General, Department of Health and Human Servces. 1993. *State Medical Boards and Quality-of-Care Cases: Promising Approaches*. Boston: Office of Inspector General, 5.

116. J. L. Fink. 1994. *Pharmacy Law Digest* (Media, PA: Harwal): NABP Survey of Pharmacy Law, A-50s.

117. Iowa Code Ann. § 145.3(3)(b).

118. M. H. Epstein and B. S. Kurtzig. 1994. "Statewide Health Information: A Tool for Improving Hospital Accountability." *Joint Commission Journal on Quality Improvement* 20 (7): 370.

119. Programs are already being developed for computerized review of claims data, medical records, or both, to analyze quality of care. See D. W. Garnick, J. Fowles, A. G. Lawthers, J. P. Weiner, S. T. Parente, and H. R. Palmer. 1994. "Focus on Quality: Profiling Physicians' Practice Patterns." *Journal of Ambulatory Care Management*, 17 (3): 44; D. W. Garnick, A. G. Lawthers, R. H. Palmer, S. J. R. Moentmann, J. Fowles, and J. P. Weiner. 1994. "A Computerized System for Reviewing Medical Records from Physicians' Offices." *Joint Commission Journal on Quality Improvement* 20 (12): 679; J. P. Weiner, N. R. Power, D. Steinwachs, and G. Dent. 1990. "Applying Insurance Claims Data to Assess Quality of Care." *Quality Review Bulletin* 16 (12): 424.

120. Some boards already do this. See Inspector General, *Promising Approaches*, 8.

121. Ibid., 9.

122. Ibid., 10–11; See "Call for Medical Experts Brings Gratifying Response." *Action Report, Medical Board of California* (April 1995): 1.

123. See Office of Inspector General, Department of Health and Human Services. 1990. *Quality Assurance Activities of Medical Licensure Authorities in the United States and Canada*. Boston: Office of Inspector General, A-2.

124. 1996. "Disciplinary Issues Stretch State Medical Board Resources." *State Health Notes* 17 (221): 1.

125. Inspector General, *Promising Approaches*, 7.

126. Ibid., 21.

127. Ibid., 11.

128. See W. D. Dauphinee. 1995. "Assessing Clinical Performance: Where Do We Stand and What Might We Expect." *Journal of the American Medical Association* 274 (9): 741; C. H. McGuire. 1995. "Reflections of a Maverick Measurement Maven." *Journal of the American Medical Association* 274 (9): 735; D. Langsley.

1991. "Medical Competence and Performance Assessment: A New Era," *Journal of the American Medical Association* 266 (7): 977 (discussing new approaches to performance assessment). See also D. J. Klass. 1991. "Standardized Patients in Clinical Skills Assessment: Experience at Southern Illinois University and the University of Manitoba." *Federation Bulletin* 78 (2): 35.

129. G. R. Norman, D. A. Davis, S. Lamb, E. Hanna, P. Caulford, and T. Kaigas. 1993. "Competency Assessment of Primary Care Physicians as Part of a Peer Review Program." *Journal of the American Medical Association* 270 (9): 1046; Inspector General, *Quality Assurance*, B-5–B-7.

130. Rettie, "Evaluating."

131. See Inspector General, *Quality Assurance*, A-3 (describing the California Board's Practice).

132. See *Smith v. Board of Medical Quality Assurance*, 248 Cal. Rptr. 704 (Cal. App. 1988).

133. Inspector General, *Promising Approaches*, 17.

134. Ibid., 17–20.

135. See F. Rosner, J. A. Balint, and R. M. Stein. 1994. "Remedial Medical Education." *Archives of Internal Medicine* 145 (3) 274.

136. See R. S. Walzer and S. Miltimore. 1993. "Mandated Supervision, Monitoring, and Therapy of Disciplined Health Care Professionals." *The Journal of Legal Medicine* 14 (4): 565.

137. See Inspector General, *Quality Assurance*, A-3–A-4; Inspector General, *Promising Approaches*, 22; T. C. Meyer. 1990. "The Role of the Remedial CME." *Federation Bulletin* 77 (6): 182, describing remedial CME programs sponsored by state medical boards.

138. Inspector General, *Promising Approaches*, 22.

139. Finnocchio, *Reforming Health Care*, 25.

140. Ibid., 25–56.

141. See D. A. Davis, M. A. Thompson, A. D. Oxman, and B. Haynes. 1995. "Changing Physician Performance: A Systematic Review of the Effect of Continuing Medical Education Strategies." *Journal of the American Medical Association* 274 (9): 700.

142. See L. Oberman. 1995. "Retesting, Time Limits Recurring Credential Plans." *American Medical News* 37 (13): 3.

143. See Citizens Advocacy Center. 1995. *The Role of Licensing in Assuring the Continued Competency of Health Care Professionals*. Washington, DC: Citizens Advocacy Center.

144. As of 1994, 19 of the 24 boards had committed themselves to mandatory recertification. See E. L. Mancall and P. G. Bashook. 1994. *Recertification: New Evaluation Methods and Strategies*. Evanston, IL: American Board of Medical Specialties, xi.

145. Citizen Advocacy Center and National Council of State Boards of Nursing. 1996. *Crafting Public Protection for the 21st Century: The Role of Nursing Regulation*. Chicago: National Council of State Boards of Nursing, 19.

146. Citizens Advocacy Center. 1995. *The Role of Licensing in Assuring the Continuing Competence of Health Care Professionals*. Washington, DC: Citizens Advocacy Center, 9.

147. See L. B. Buckler. 1995. "Medical Licensure in the 21st Century: Are We Ready?" *Federation Bulletin* 82 (4): 203.

148. This was the approach recommended by New York's Advisory Committee on Periodic Physician Recredentialing. See A. Gellhorn. 1991. "Periodic Physician Recredentialing." *Journal of the American Medical Association* 265 (6): 752.

149. Mancall and Bashook, *Recertification*.

150. See Brennan and Berwick, *New Rules*, 374–75, 381–84.

151. See S. McIlrath. 1994. "Board-Certified Only Need Apply." *American Medical News* 37 (46): 1.

REGULATORY RESPONSES TO PROFESSIONAL MISCONDUCT: SEXUAL MISCONDUCT, CONTROLLED SUBSTANCES, AND IMPAIRMENT

Sandra Johnson

THE TYPICAL health professional licensure statute includes a substantial list of specific grounds for discipline. Among the common grounds for discipline relating to physicians are conviction of a felony relating to the attributes necessary for the practice of the profession, unlawful sale of drugs, and aiding and abetting the unauthorized practice of medicine.[1] Some states have enacted more unusual grounds for discipline, including willful failure to comply with statutory informed consent requirements for sterilization procedures; prescribing, dispensing, administering, or furnishing liquid silicone breast implants; and violating statutory restrictions on the use of laetrile.[2]

This chapter focuses on three of the most prominent grounds for professional disciplinary intervention: sexual misconduct, inappropriate prescription of controlled substances, and impairment due to substance abuse. The issue of sexual activity with patients has generated a disproportionate number of appellate cases and continues to attract considerable attention from the public and the profession. Sanctions for prescriptive practices relating to controlled substances have come under scrutiny for their effect on the undertreatment of pain. Impairment due to substance abuse forms the basis of the majority of disciplinary actions. Impairment is also of interest because it is often addressed through alternative procedures other than the enforcement-oriented disciplinary process, and because it raises significant disability discrimination issues.

Sexual Misconduct

Estimates of the percentage of physicians who have had sexual activity with patients vary, ranging from five to ten percent of practicing physicians, although some view these estimates as understated.[3] In a survey of 10,000 physicians, producing a response rate of approximately 19 percent, 10 percent of male physicians and 4 percent of female physicians (totaling 9 percent of all physicians responding) reported sexual contact with one or more patients; 42 percent of those reporting any sexual contact reported sexual activity with multiple patients; and 23 percent of all responding physicians (35 percent of all responding obstetrician-gynecologists) reported that at least one of their patients had told them of sexual contact with a treating physician.[4]

Sexual misconduct is considered a major issue by medical licensure boards.[5] The incidence of disciplinary actions for sexual misconduct has increased rapidly, nearly tripling between 1990 and 1995; and medical licensure boards have been criticized for failing to effectively pursue disciplinary actions in this area.[6]

AMA Opinion

In late 1991, the House of Delegates of the AMA adopted a report of the Council on Ethical and Judicial Affairs concerning physician-patient sexual conduct. The Council concluded that "sexual contact or romantic relationship concurrent with the physician-patient relationship is unethical."[7] In justifying its conclusion, the AMA argued that the emotional engagement and power imbalance characteristic of the physician-patient relationship make any sexual contact or romantic relationship unethical, even that to which the patient may have consented. The Council's report explained that sexual activity and "romantic interactions" may "detract from the goals of the physician-patient relationship" and may "obscure the physician's objective judgment concerning the patient's healthcare." But the opinion does not limit the prohibition on sexual activity to situations in which such a negative outcome has in fact occurred. Nor does the opinion provide an exemption or exclusion for behavior claimed to be the subject of mutual consent. In setting the irrebuttable presumption that all physician-patient sexual activity is unethical, the AMA has extended arguments that have supported a long-standing ban on therapist-patient sexual activity in the psychotherapeutic context[8] to all physician-patient contexts.[9]

The ethical characterization of sexual activity between a physician and a former patient is more controversial. In a survey in which 94 percent of doctors stated that they opposed sexual contact with current patients, only 37 percent considered sexual contact with former patients unacceptable.[10] The 1991 Opinion of the AMA Council states that the minimum duty of a physician in cases in which a "true romantic relationship" develops is to terminate the professional relationship. The Opinion states that subsequent sexual activity may still be unethical under particular circumstances. However, even in the case of psychotherapists, where ethical and legal prohibitions against sexual activity with current patients are long-standing, sexual activity with former patients is not viewed as invariably unethical.[11]

Disciplinary Standards

State professional boards are authorized to take disciplinary action in cases of sexual misconduct either under generic statutory disciplinary grounds or under more specific statutory prohibitions against sexual activity with patients or former patients. Healthcare professionals engaging in sexual activity with patients or former patients may also be subject to claims for malpractice or to prosecution for criminal conduct under general sexual assault statutes[12] or under more recent statutes specifically categorizing sexual activity with patients as criminal.[13] In most states, conviction of a crime, at least one that relates to the attributes required for the practice of the profession, also forms an independent ground for discipline;[14] thus, the professional who is convicted of sexual assault of a patient may face disciplinary action as a result of that conviction.[15] Discipline for sexual misconduct with patients satisfies the constitutional requirement[16] that licensure standards must rationally relate to fitness or capacity to practice.[17]

General statutory grounds for discipline, such as "unprofessional conduct" or "moral turpitude," can provide the basis for discipline of healthcare professionals engaging in sexual relations with patients. These general disciplinary terms have been challenged as being unconstitutionally vague in their application to instances of sexual activity between healthcare professionals and patients, but those challenges have failed.[18] Vagueness challenges have also been brought against the prosecution of physicians under sexual assault statutes. In *People v. Burpo*,[19] for example, the Illinois Supreme Court held that the general sexual assault statute was not unconstitutionally vague in its application to a gynecologist accused of sexual assault in the conduct of physical examinations. The court held that the prosecution must prove that the gynecologist knew that the patient did not consent (with an assumption that patient consent reaches only examinations that are reasonable in nature) and that the gynecologist "possessed a mental state of intent, knowledge, or recklessness."

Several states have enacted specific disciplinary statutes prohibiting sexual relations with patients. Current statutes specifically addressing sexual activity with current or former patients do not necessarily mirror the scope of the AMA Council Opinion, however. For example, some states proscribe "exercising influence" for the purpose of engaging in sexual activity.[20] Others penalize only sexual contact that is exploitative of the physician-patient relationship.[21] These statutes would appear to require specific proof of exploitation and advantage-taking, while the Council Opinion establishes an irrebuttable presumption of exploitation for evaluating the ethical character of such activity. The AMA does not intend the Council's Opinions to have the force of law, and it may be justifiable to draw legal proscriptions more narrowly than ethical standards. Still, the AMA position should influence agencies and courts in the evaluation of individual cases.[22]

Statutes that specifically penalize only sexual activity with "patients" may be interpreted fairly as not reaching sexual activity with former patients. In *Haley v. Medical Disciplinary Board*,[23] the court held that a statutory prohibition against "sexual contact with a patient" did not reach sexual activity between a surgeon and his 16-year-old former patient, even though the activity occurred in close proximity to the relationship. The court held, however, that the disciplinary agency could proceed under more general disciplinary standards relating to moral turpitude.

Statutes specifically prohibiting sexual contact with former patients often take a bright-line approach, characterizing as grounds for discipline sexual relationships that occur within a particular time frame after the termination of the professional relationship.[24] In contrast, the AMA standard requires close examination of the parties' relationship on an individual case-by-case basis and states that sexual activity with former patients is unethical if "sexual contact occurred as a result of the use or exploitation of trust, knowledge, influence, or emotions derived from the former professional relationship."

Proving the continued existence or termination of the professional-patient relationship raises difficult factual issues. In *Haley*, for example, the court identified cases in which a physician-patient relationship may be more likely to exist over some time, specifically distinguishing oncologists, internists, family physicians, and psychiatrists from surgeons. In *Heinecke v. Department of Commerce*,[25] the Utah Court of Appeals found a continuing professional relationship where a nurse who had provided nursing care to an institutionalized patient with multiple personality disorder continued to assist in the care of the patient after discharge but without compensation. The court held that the nursing board had authority to discipline because the nurse-patient relationship had not been definitely and clearly terminated and that the nurse had taken advantage of knowledge gained in the course of the professional relationship.[26]

The prosecution of disciplinary actions for sexual misconduct often raises issues concerning the relative credibility of the professional and patient as to what occurred between them. Courts generally rely on the findings of the trier of fact as to credibility in these cases,[27] just as they generally do in review of disciplinary actions.[28] State licensing boards responding to a survey reported the use of expert testimony in limited cases to address specific issues of credibility, including credibility questions raised by a patient's substantial delay in filing a complaint and evaluation of the complainant's psychiatric history as it may have affected the complaint.[29] Empirical research indicates that delays in reporting by patients may be due to emotional and emotion-related physical injuries similar to those suffered by the victims of sexual assault[30] or to referral of the patient by the offending professional to physicians sympathetic to the professional.[31] The Federation of State Medical Boards has issued a report establishing guidelines for the conduct of investigations and hearings related to instances of sexual misconduct that take account of the psychological context.[32]

Controlled Substances and Pain Relief

Disciplinary actions related to the prescription of controlled substances dominate the activity of state medical licensure boards. Disciplinary agencies are concerned with impaired physicians who self-prescribe controlled substances or divert drugs to their own use.[33] Agencies want to exclude from practice physicians who are fraudulent or incompetent in their prescriptive practices, presenting a physical or financial threat to their patients by prescribing controlled substances when they are believed to be ineffective or dangerous.[34] State disciplinary boards are also involved, often at the insistence of or in collaboration with criminal prosecutors, in the "war on drugs," penalizing physicians who inappropriately prescribe controlled substances that may be diverted to "street use" or who are in fact "drug dealers" themselves, abusing their prescriptive authority.[35] Disciplinary action against physicians for their prescriptive practices relating to controlled substances has another side, however.

The number of patients who suffer undertreated and needless pain in the United States is high. Surveys indicate that at least 40 percent of white, male cancer patients experience untreated pain. Further, the incidence of undertreatment relates to gender, race, disability, and age, with the elderly and children, women and minorities at the highest risk for medical neglect of pain relief.[36] In one survey, one-third of physicians reported intentionally undermedicating for pain.[37] Physicians report that they undertreat for pain in part from fear of legal penalties, especially disciplinary action.[38]

Physicians' fears of disciplinary action are not unfounded. There is some evidence, for example, that many state medical boards have not integrated the more current approaches to the use of controlled substances in pain management within their disciplinary processes and may mischaracterize acceptable dosage and length-of-treatment practices as inappropriate and illegitimate.[39] In addition, the prosecutorial stance stimulated by the war on drugs heightens the punitive character of investigations and may unintentionally interfere with adequate pain relief as physicians steer well clear of practices that may trigger inquiry.[40] Increasing scrutiny of the effectiveness of disciplinary agencies in protecting the public may have a similar effect. Finally, reported case law involving review of disciplinary actions against physicians for their prescriptive practices reveals that the medical licensure boards have not been entirely successful in distinguishing between "good doctors" who are providing effective medication to patients experiencing pain, and "bad doctors" who are providing controlled substances to patients who do not need the medication.

Screening for Bad Practices

A central issue in effective discipline for inappropriate prescription of controlled substances is distinguishing appropriate from inappropriate practices. In this, disciplinary action for inappropriate prescription of controlled substances takes on some of the characteristics of disciplinary action for incompetence, an area that has presented agencies with continuing challenges.[41]

Enforcement efforts have used the sheer volume of prescriptions, measured in terms of frequency of prescriptions or dosages or polypharmacy per patient or across the physician's entire patient population, as a major indicator of inappropriate use. Investigative and disciplinary practices have allowed for a greater margin for doctors who are treating terminal patients or patients with cancer pain. Such a margin benefits those patients and their physicians, but is not responsive to the many patients who have chronic, nonmalignant pain.

Volume indicators standing alone can cast the net too widely, capturing physicians who are legitimately treating large numbers of patients for pain or patients with long-term intractable pain. If volume indicators are viewed as a screening test, it may be thought that the use of such an overly sensitive test is here justifiable. The effect, however, of using prescribing volume as a trigger for investigation appears to be to chill doctors in their treatment of patients in pain, resulting in turn in medical neglect and unnecessary suffering. The fact that disciplinary action may not be pursued to completion or is overturned on appeal is not consoling to physicians who are subject to investigative and disciplinary scrutiny that tends to be punitive and quasi-criminal in nature.[42]

In *Hollabaugh v. Arkansas State Medical Board*,[43] for example, Dr. Hollabaugh appealed sanctions levied by the board for her prescriptive practices relating to controlled substances. The only testimony provided against Dr. Hollabaugh was the testimony of the board's investigator, a pharmacist, who testified only as to the "types, amounts, and frequency" of Hollabaugh's prescriptions. The board had placed Dr. Hollabaugh's license on probation for one year, required 50 hours of CME on pain management, ordered her to refrain from prescribing Schedule II and Schedule III drugs, and required her to be monitored by the state's pharmacy board. The trial court affirmed.

The court of appeals reversed, however, holding that the board's decision was not supported by substantial evidence on the record. Dr. Hollabaugh testified about her reasons for the prescriptions providing, in the court's view, "much detail about [her patients'] medical condition." She testified as well that she believed that pain was seriously undertreated. The record did not support the board's action, according to the court, because it did not contain expert testimony as to the accepted standard of practice for patients such as those treated by Hollabaugh. The Arkansas Supreme Court had established the requirement of expert testimony in disciplinary actions relating to malpractice and negligence in an earlier case.[44]

It is likely that volume screens or red flags will continue to play some role in the enforcement process. Serious adjustments have to be made, however, in the use of such data in individual cases in the investigation process as well as at the disciplinary stage.[45]

Requiring expert testimony is a good first step to correcting uninformed board actions. The expert, however, should be especially qualified in the treatment of pain if current and emerging state-of-the-art standards are to be available as a defense to physicians treating patients for pain. Not all physicians are qualified to testify concerning prescriptive practices. For example, the court in *Hoover v. Agency for Health Care Administration*[46] overturned disciplinary action against the licensee because the board's two "experts" had no experience in treating chronic pain patients and had not been provided with the medical records of the patients at issue.

Other indicators of bad prescriptive practices include the physician's failure to follow customary diagnostic and documentation processes. Physician failure to perform a physical examination or take the medical history of a patient, failure to maintain accurate and current medical records on each patient, failure to attempt to diagnose the underlying condition causing pain, and failure to document a treatment plan or monitor patients on a regular basis over the long term is likely to be viewed as proof of illegitimate prescriptive practices. The courts have frequently used these minimal requirements of competent medical practice as a basis for review of disciplinary or criminal action against physicians for their prescriptive practices.[47] These indicators are generally supportable and screen effectively for the more egregious violators. They require a review of the physician's patient records, however, and therefore do subject the physician to investigation.

Standards for Pain Management

The absence of established medical standards for prescriptive practices in the treatment of pain in many circumstances presents a second difficult issue for the disciplinary process. Medical standards for the use of controlled substances in pain management are changing drastically. Basic assumptions underlying restrictive professional practices, such as fear of addiction of terminal patients, blanket disapproval of long-term use of controlled substances, and fear of fatal side effects, have been undercut with increased research and the evolution of pain control as a specialty.

Practice guidelines on pain management for certain conditions, particularly for the treatment of acute pain and cancer pain, have been developed recently[48] and boards should make reference to them.[49] Consensus on the treatment of chronic pain is still elusive, however.

This lack of consensus has implications for the disciplinary process and for judicial review of disciplinary actions. In *In the Matter of DiLeo*,[50] the court reviewed the testimony of the prosecution's chief witness, who testified that the duration of treatment with controlled substances was excessive. The court noted that the expert "admitted . . . that there are no written standards published, and that there are "various schools of medical thought" concerning how long patients with chronic pain may be treated with controlled substances. The court correctly was not persuaded by the expert's testimony that the professional standard of care was established by the Physician's Desk Reference (PDR). The PDR indicated that the prescribed drugs were intended for short-term use only. The court held that the board's sanctions against DiLeo were not supported by substantial evidence.

Lack of consensus may not always be determinative, however. In *People v. Schade*,[51] the California Court of Appeals reviewed expert testimony from ten experts concerning the prescriptive practices of Dr. Schade. The court's opinion details the conflicting testimony of the witnesses concerning the use of controlled substances for chronic noncancer pain. Several of the experts had testified that long-term use of narcotics is categorically inappropriate for chronic noncancer pain, and several had testified that such use is appropriate. The court recognized the conflict over acceptable standards for treatment of chronic pain, but in the end concluded that there was a "plethora of evidence" that the physician had "failed to make any attempt" to treat the patients except by prescribing controlled substances. It cited evidence that the physician routinely failed to examine the patients physically, failed to take medical histories, did not perform diagnostic or monitoring lab tests, and did not refer patients to specialists.

Chemically Dependent Patients

Enforcement and regulatory activity have been particularly concerned with the prescription of controlled substances for patients who are chemically dependent. States commonly have specific statutory restrictions relating to such patients. Chemically dependent or drug-dependent patients are thought to be more likely to divert drugs to illegal uses. Those patients who become addicted to or dependent upon prescription pain relievers during the course of treatment are viewed as more likely to be exploited by their physicians or to suffer serious physical harm from the physician's failure to monitor their conditions. Drug-dependent individuals may seek out physicians as an alternative source to the street trade. Punitive regulatory action in relation to drug-dependent patients presents two difficulties, however.[52]

First, patients who are drug dependent may experience severe pain unrelated to their drug addiction, as they are equally or at times more likely to contract painful diseases such as acquired immunodeficiency syndrome (AIDS) or cancer. Using their preexisting addiction as a justification to deny adequate treatment of intractable pain punishes them because of their status and causes avoidable suffering. Second, there is either lack of consensus or broad misunderstanding over the appropriate definition of the state of drug dependency or drug addiction. Diagnosis of addiction may depend on the specialty and background of the diagnostician, with pain specialists and addictionologists reaching different conclusions.[53] Patients who have used controlled substances in the legitimate effort to control chronic pain—even patients who have terminal cancer and use controlled substances in large quantities—have been viewed as addicts, though that view certainly does not conform to current standards of practice.[54]

In *People v. Schade* (discussed above), the defendant challenged his convictions for prescribing controlled substances for "addicts." The issue presented on appeal was whether the trial court was required to instruct the jury on the meaning of the term "addict." In its opinion, the California Court of Appeals provided a lengthy discussion of the statutory provision restricting treatment with controlled substances of an "addict" or "habitual user." The court concluded that "addict" is a technical term rather than one that is commonly understood, and that its definition was essential to the defendant's conviction for violation of that section of the statute.

The court reviewed the testimony of nine experts as to the meaning of addiction. The court commented that there was "an abundance of definitions of addiction given to the jury" by the experts and that the nine experts "could not all agree upon a single acceptable definition."

The court's discussion of the way jurors might interpret the term addict is instructive regarding the legal implications of this dispute:

> The jurors could have disagreed about what addiction meant but have decided that if a patient met any definition of addict then the patient was an addict. Thus, one juror might have believed a patient was an addict because the patient engaged in drug-seeking behavior even though that juror did not believe the patient was psychologically or physically dependent. Another juror might have believed a patient was psychologically dependent. A third juror might have decided the patient was physically dependent. A fourth juror might have believed the patient had developed a tolerance for the drug but was not psychologically or physically dependent, and so on. Thus, it is conceivable that not defining "addict" for the jury . . . made it easier for appellant to be convicted.

The court found that statutory definitions of "addict" failed to provide a consistent definition of the term. The court defined addiction as the sum of "three characteristic mental and physical responses of the addiction process: i.e., emotional dependence, tolerance, and physical dependence."[55]

Statutes and Policies

Some state medical boards are responding to the problem of regulatory discouragement of the adequate treatment of pain. Some boards have adopted policies that specifically state that controlled substances are appropriate for the management of pain.[56] The best known of these efforts is the "Pain Summit" undertaken by the State of California.[57]

Some states have adopted specific "intractable pain statutes" that are intended to encourage the provision of effective pain relief by stating that the use of controlled substances is acceptable for pain management or by providing physicians immunity or some other level of protection from disciplinary action.[58] These statutes vary widely among the states.[59]

Some reach only physicians.[60] Physicians' fears and behaviors have attracted the most public attention. Many more professionals have prescriptive authority, however, and care for patients in pain.[61] In addition, pharmacists are subject to even more scrutiny, in particular by federal enforcement agencies,[62] and pharmacist practices also affect patients' access to controlled substances.[63]

Some of the state statutes do not protect the physician from disciplinary action if the patient is drug dependent.[64] Failure to include the treatment of chemically dependent patients is undesirable for the reasons discussed earlier.

A few of these states simply provide that a physician may prescribe controlled substances for the treatment of pain so long as the physician does so within accepted medical standards. As discussed above, however, part of the current problem is that accepted medical standards are nonexistent for some conditions and evolving for others.[65]

At least one statute requires the patient's written consent to pain medication.[66] On the other hand, a few states prohibit healthcare facilities from restricting the use of controlled substances for the treatment of pain.[67]

There is heightened awareness of the negative effect of disciplinary action for the prescription of controlled substances for the treatment of pain. Though evolving and inadequate standards of practice complicate the entire process, a shift in emphasis that would encourage adequate pain relief is necessary.

Impairment

The response of professional boards to impairment is a third area of concern. In a survey of state medical boards, 85 percent reported that they addressed psychological conditions, physical disabilities, and age-related cognitive defects as impairments. Twenty percent reported addressing sexual misconduct as a question of impairment.[68] The inclusion of "sexual misconduct" among the categories of impairment is troubling because it implies that an act or behavior that is quite harmful to patients and may be criminal is an "impairment." The Federation of State Medical Boards has taken the position that sexual misconduct is not an impairment and, further, that "although a mental disorder may be a basis for sexual misconduct, . . . sexual misconduct usually is not caused by physical/mental impairment." The Committee also stated that "sexual addiction," although a commonly used phrase, is not recognized as a disease.[69]

Most cases of impairment involve substance abuse. Estimates of the incidence of physician dependency on drugs and alcohol vary. One survey of physicians reported that 7.9 percent of responding physicians stated that they were chemically dependent at some time in their lives and that 2.1 percent stated that they were chemically dependent during the previous year. Over 9 percent of responding physicians reported having five or more drinks in one day at least once in the past month, with .6 percent reporting five or more drinks daily. The survey also found that doctors were less likely than the general population to use illicit drugs. Because of their prescriptive authority, however, there was a high rate of self-medication with controlled substances, ranging from 11.4 to 17.6 percent depending on the drug.[70] Another study of physicians under the age of forty reported that 38 percent of physicians in that age group reported continued use of marijuana, cocaine, and other drugs, and 42 percent reported treating themselves with mind-affecting drugs in the year prior to the survey.[71] Estimates of chemical dependency among nurses hover around six to seven percent.[72]

Many studies report that physicians do not differ from the general population, adjusted for socioeconomic characteristics, in their use of alcohol and some drugs,[73] although the level of alcohol abuse may reach 12 to 14 percent among both physicians and the general population.[74] Some physicians, however, may be at a greater risk of chemical dependency. For example, groups with higher rates of dependency include anesthesiologists, family and general practitioners, academicians, smokers, and those with a family history of dependency.[75]

Impairment due to drug or alcohol is a common ground for professional discipline.[76] The percentage of doctors sanctioned by or participating in rehabilitation programs sponsored within state licensing systems is estimated to range from one to three percent, causing the authors of one study to observe that the "survey estimates . . . suggest a higher rate of physician abuse or dependence than these cumulative estimates from state programs."[77] Physicians and other healthcare professionals who use alcohol and drugs are not necessarily impaired, however.[78]

Defining and Detecting Impairment

A threshold issue in the relationship of the disciplinary system to the impaired professional is the definition of what constitutes prohibited conduct. Statutory provisions generally require that the professional's use of drugs or alcohol result in some impairment in the professional's ability to practice medicine with reasonable skill, care, and safety in order to form a basis for discipline or other intervention.[79] Others require that the use of drugs or alcohol present a danger to the public or to the licensee.[80] Mere use or dependency, standing alone, would not be sufficient for disciplinary action under such statutes, although some courts in the past have been willing to go to considerable lengths in assuming impairment from dependency.[81] Statutes that allow discipline where the professional is impaired or presents a danger do not require the board to prove actual injury to any individual patient, of course, but they would require some evidence that the physician's condition presents increased risk of harm.[82]

Some statutes governing disciplinary action for the use of alcohol or drugs require only that the professional be "addicted," "dependent," or a "habitual user" of the substances.[83] The use of terms such as addiction and dependency in such statutes is subject to the same definitional disputes that were reviewed in the prior section on prescription of controlled substances.[84] Other issues also are raised in the context of discipline. In *Mississippi State Board of Nursing v. Wilson*,[85] the court considered the discipline imposed on a nurse who had been treated for "cocaine addiction," who had stolen controlled substances from his employer, and who had been disciplined previously for related behaviors. At the time of sanction, the nurse had not used drugs for over a year. The nursing board argued that the nurse's behavior in years past constituted evidence that the nurse was addicted or dependent. The court rejected this argument and held that the terms required proof of "ongoing and continuous use" and not "isolated instances of usage." The court held that the statute required active addiction, rather than a past record of addiction.[86]

In comparison, in *Burns v. Board of Nursing*,[87] the Supreme Court of Iowa concluded that several indications of intoxication in work settings were adequate in themselves to support the board's finding that the nurse was a habitual user and subject to discipline under the statute, even though the incidents were not continuous. Statutes providing that dependency or habitual use standing alone support discipline may present a difficulty under the Americans with Disabilities Act (discussed below) depending on their interpretation.

The detection and investigation of cases of potential impairment also present legal issues relating to the board's authority to compel mental and physical examinations of licensees. On the first level, the authority of the board to compel examinations is bounded by the authority granted in the licensure statute.[88] Second, state or federal constitutional concerns limit compulsory physical and mental exams. Rights to privacy and due process and freedom from unreasonable search and seizure will apply in such cases. In general terms, constitutional constraints require that the state's interest in protecting the public be balanced with the individual's interests and that the intrusion upon the individual's interests be as limited as possible. In applying this balancing test to specific cases, courts have found that conducting the exam in a location that would not subject the licensee to excess scrutiny and maintaining confidentiality of the records of the exam were important. This balancing test may also restrict the board's ability to compel multiple examinations.[89]

Impaired Professional Programs

Most states have established programs to provide rehabilitative, non-punitive interventions for impaired nurses, physicians, and other health professionals.[90] The rehabilitative approach to impairment naturally emerges from the understanding of chemical dependency, especially in professionals, as an illness rather than a failure in character. It also responds to perceived concerns that a punitive disciplinary approach pushes impaired healthcare providers undercover, risking greater injury to the public. It is hoped that the availability of a program of nonpunitive rehabilitation encourages a higher rate of reporting and self-reporting of impaired professionals.[91] A focus on rehabilitation rather than punishment may be meeting more resistance in discipline of nurses as compared to physicians.[92]

Impaired physician programs (IPPs) are structured differently among the states.[93] Some are wholly voluntary with no threat of referral to disciplinary authorities, while others are coercive or board mandated, with discipline held in abeyance as long as the doctor participates in the program of rehabilitation; and still other programs allow admission of physicians falling into each category.[94]

There are several issues that arise in the administration of such programs and in the relations between these diversion programs and the boards themselves. The Federation of State Medical Boards issued a policy statement in 1995 that describes a model IPP from the perspective of the boards.[95] The issues addressed in this policy statement relate to continuing tension between rehabilitation efforts and protection of the public from impaired physicians.

The Federation's model requires that the board operate the program under its own auspices or directly contract with another organization. The Federation's model encourages substantial interaction between the disciplinary board and the IPP. It assumes that participation may be either voluntary or board mandated, although early efforts with diversion programs questioned nonvoluntary participation.[96] Although the Federation's policy document recognizes that confidentiality is important to encouraging voluntary participation in the IPP, the Federation recommends that the IPP notify a board staff member (as opposed to a board member) of the identity of all participating physicians and that the IPP be required to notify the medical board formally in the case of noncompliance. Again, this is a controversial provision. In *Kees v. Medical Board of California*,[97] however, the court held that the physician must be a "formal" participant in the diversion program in order to be shielded from disciplinary action.

Relapse is a significant issue for IPP programs. Estimates of the incidence of relapse vary, but some percentage is always expected. Some studies of physician treatment programs indicate relapse rates of 10 to 20 percent,[98] with one estimating that 10 percent of participants fail and are referred for disciplinary action.[99] Other studies indicate relapse rates ranging from 30 to 57 percent, though the severity and duration of relapse may vary.[100]

Americans with Disabilities Act

"Impairment" is a term of art in professional licensure; but it is also a central term in the federal Americans with Disabilities Act (ADA),[101] which prohibits discrimination against persons who have a physical or mental impairment or a record of such impairment or are viewed as having such an impairment.[102] A finding of impairment has a radically different result under each of these statutes: for the licensure statute, an impairment requires discipline involving removal from or limitation in practice; but for the ADA, an impairment triggers statutory protection and allows the individual to claim rights under the Act (though perhaps not his or her license in the end).

Title II of the ADA applies to the licensing functions of the professional licensure boards of the states.[103] The Act reaches the application, examination, and admission functions as well as the disciplinary functions, including the boards' impaired physician programs.[104] Title II of the Act is enforced by the U.S. Department of Justice and through private suits brought by individuals.[105] Claimants under Title II of the ADA are not required to exhaust administrative remedies prior to filing suit. The 1990 Act is relatively new, and there has been little litigation concerning the application of the Act to these functions. Case law developed under the earlier federal Rehabilitation Act, however, is applicable to the interpretation of the ADA.

ADA analysis under Title II first requires that the individual licensee be disabled within the terms of the Act. The definition of disability requires that the person have an impairment that limits major life activities or have a record of or be perceived to have such an impairment.[106] It covers both physical and mental disorders, as well as specific learning disabilities.

Most of the activity in physician impairment programs and discipline relates to the abuse of drugs and alcohol. Alcoholism is not addressed in Title II. It may be assumed that alcoholism either is an impairment or is viewed as an impairment so that individuals who are alcoholics do fall within the protection of the Act. As discussed below, however, the alcoholic must be otherwise qualified to practice.

Individuals who are illegally using drugs cannot bring employment discrimination claims against private employers under the ADA when the employer has acted on the basis of the illegal use.[107] There is no parallel statutory provision for Title II, but the Justice Department regulations provide that the Act does not prohibit discrimination based on "current" illegal use of drugs. The regulations provide, however, that the agency may not deny rehabilitation services to an individual on the basis of current illegal drug use except when that use continues during the course of the program.[108]

"Current use" is defined in the regulations as use that has "occurred recently enough to justify a reasonable belief that a person's drug use is current or a real and ongoing problem." There is a difference of opinion on the meaning of this definition.[109] The Colorado Court of Appeals has held that the ADA did not protect a physician who had ceased using drugs illegally only a short time prior to disciplinary action and who had a record of recurrent illegal drug use and presented a high risk of relapse.[110]

If a person has a disability, the next step in the analysis is to judge whether the individual is "qualified." The ADA does not require that a disabled individual be granted a license or be free from sanction simply because he or she is disabled.

The determination of whether the disabled person is "qualified" requires an assessment of the individual's abilities and of the essential requirements for practice. It also requires an evaluation of accommodations that can reasonably be made for the individual's disability without fundamentally altering the practice. Professional schools have had some experience in litigation concerning essential requirements for professional practice.[111] In such contexts, the courts have accorded the schools some deference for academic judgment. There is also some experience with the issue in relation to application and examination procedures used for professional licensure.[112]

According to the Department of Justice, licensure boards are not required to license persons who present a "direct threat to the health or safety of others" if reasonable modifications of board policies, practices, or procedures will not eliminate that risk.[113] The "direct threat" analysis will be most important to boards in disciplinary cases involving impaired physicians. Whether a practitioner poses a direct risk to health and safety requires an individualized evaluation, based on current medical evidence to determine the nature, duration, and severity of the risk; the probability that the potential injury will occur; and whether reasonable modifications will mitigate the risk. This test was established by the U.S. Supreme Court in a case involving tuberculosis, *School Board of Nassau County v. Arline*,[114] but the test is equally applicable to most physician impairments. In Arline, the Supreme Court considered the case of a teacher with tuberculosis who claimed that she was dismissed from her teaching position because her employer believed that there was a threat to the health of her students and others. The Court rejected her position that any contagiousness made the teacher an unacceptable risk and, therefore, unqualified for the job. It was in this context that the Court adopted the AMA's offer of standards to be used to assess risks of harm presented by individuals with contagious or other diseases. The requirement of a more individualized assessment requires that the boards operate on more than assumptions and stereotypes about specific disabilities, including chemical dependency and mental disorders. Data-based decisions and expert evaluations will be important.

Early cases indicate some latitude for board actions in the context of discipline. For example, in *Alexander v. Margolis*,[115] the federal trial court held that the physician was not "qualified" and that the ADA did not prohibit disciplinary action against him. The doctor had been convicted and imprisoned for violation of federal drug law but claimed that his behavior was due to his bipolar disorder. The board stated in its findings of fact that the existence of the illness was "an important aspect" of the licensee's ability, but that its refusal to reinstate the doctor's license was based on his conviction of a felony for knowingly distributing drugs. The court accorded the board substantial deference.[116] The court stated that the board must have "discretion" to protect the public, and that there would be no violation of the ADA absent an abuse of the board's discretion. The court concluded that, "given the physician's necessary independence to practice," no reasonable modification could be made to the practice of restricting licensure to persons "without evidence of mental disabilities." The court stated this too broadly, and it is likely that distinctions will be made in later cases relating to different types of mental impairments. Further, mental disorders (and physical disabilities) are not relevant to licensure unless they affect the individual's ability to practice medicine.

In contrast, the federal district court in *Medical Society of New Jersey v. Jacobs*[117] set a boundary on the court's deference to professional licensure boards by requiring that the board more narrowly focus its actions on behavior that affects the ability to practice medicine. The court reviewed the state's application process for licensure and found that questions relating to the applicant's history of mental illness and counseling did not address behavior or the capacity to practice medicine and so violated the ADA. The court concluded that the inquiry placed "extra burdens" on certain applicants in the form of prelicensure investigation and amounted to discriminatory treatment. The case makes clear that actions short of denial, revocation, suspension, reprimand, and the like may trigger ADA concerns. Investigations, in the court's view, may be discriminatory. Required enrollment in diversion programs would seem to be similar in nature.

It is possible that courts will distinguish between admission cases and disciplinary cases and allow the boards broader latitude in discipline. At least in discipline cases, there usually is evidence of misconduct or malpractice or increased risk, and the courts have nearly uniformly ruled that the licensee is not qualified to practice in such cases.[118] Exclusion from the profession does not violate the ADA if the licensee is not qualified to practice and no reasonable accommodations can be made.

Conclusion

This review of some of the issues presented in disciplinary action for sexual misconduct, prescriptive practices regarding controlled substances, and impairment illustrates the interaction between federal law, national professional organizations (in their establishment of ethical and practice guidelines), and the state disciplinary agencies. It also provides a window into the complexity of changing standards and values facing professional disciplinary agencies as they deal with professional conduct.

Notes

1. For an overview of disciplinary procedures and grounds for disciplinary action, see B. R. Furrow, T. L. Greaney, S. H. Johnson, T. S. Jost, and R. L. Schwartz. 1995. *Health Law* §§ 3-9–3-25 St. Paul, MN: West Publishing Co.

2. Each of these is a provision of the California medical licensure statute. West's Ann. Cal. Bus. & Prof. Code §§ 2250, 2251, and 2258.

3. Council on Ethical and Judicial Affairs. 1991. "Sexual Misconduct in the Practice of Medicine." *Journal of the American Medical Association* 266 (Nov. 20): 2741.

4. N. Gartrell, N. Milliken, W. H. Goodson III, S. Thiemann, and B. Lo. 1992. "Physician-Patient Sexual Contact: Prevalence and Problems." *Western Journal of Medicine* 157 (August): 139.

5. R. P. Reaves. 1993. "Sexual Intimacies with Patients: The Regulatory Issue of the Nineties." *Federation Bulletin* 80 (Summer): 83.

6. Council on Ethical and Judicial Affairs, "Sexual Misconduct."

7. Opinions of the Council on Ethical and Judicial Affairs § 8.14 (1992).

8. On psychotherapist-patient sexual contact, see L. Jorgenson, R. Randles, and L. Strasburger. 1991. "The Furor over Psychotherapist-Patient Sexual Contact: New Solutions to an Old Problem." *William and Mary Law Review* 32: 645, and *Simmons v. United States*, 805 F.2d 1363 (9th Cir. 1986).

9. H. R. Searight and D. C. Campbell. 1993. "Physician-Patient Sexual Contact: Ethical and Legal Issues and Clinical Guidelines." *Federation Bulletin* 80 (Winter): 247, addressing primary care physicians.

10. N. Gartrell et al., "Physician-Patient Sexual Contact."

11. See, e.g., P. S. Appelbaum and L. Jorgenson. 1991. "Psychotherapist-Patient Sexual Contact after Termination of Treatment: An Analysis and a Proposal." *American Journal of Psychiatry* 148 (November): 1466. See also 740 ILCS 104/1 (1995), providing that a former patient has a cause of action against a therapist for sexual contact occurring within one year of terminating therapy.

12. See, e.g., *People of the State of Illinois v. Burpo*, 647 N.E.2d 996 (Ill. 1995).

13. L. Jorgenson et al., "The Furor." Criminal statutes specifically applying to sexual activity between physician or psychotherapist and patient include Mich. Comp. Laws Ann. § 750.520b(1)(f)(iv) (West 1984) (applicable to physicians); Minn. Stat. Ann. § 609.342(1)(g) (West 1993) (applicable to physicians, nurses, psychologists, and social workers); and West's Ann. Cal. Bus. & Prof. Code § 729 (1995) (applicable to all licensed health professionals).

14. See, e.g., 225 ILCS 65/25 (1993).

15. See, e.g., *Pons v. Ohio State Medical Board*, 614 N.E.2d 748 (Ohio 1993); *Pundy v. Department of Professional Regulation*, 570 N.E.2d 458 (Ill. App. 1991); *Perez v. Missouri State Board of Registration for the Healing Arts*, 803 S.W.2d 160 (Mo. App. 1991).

16. See, e.g., *Biard v. State Bar of Arizona*, 401 U.S. 1, 91 S.Ct. 702, 27 L.Ed.2d 639 (1971).

17. See, e.g., *Haley v. Medical Disciplinary Board*, 818 P.2d 1062 (Wash. 1991), comparing sexual activity with patients to cases of discipline for fraud or other similar conduct. But see *Gromis v. Medical Board of California*, 10 Cal. Rptr. 2d 452 (Cal. App. 1991). See generally, T. Dobash. 1993. "Physician-Patient Sexual

Contact: The Battle Between the State and the Medical Profession." *Washington & Lee Law Review* 50: 1725.

18. *Adams. v. Texas State Board of Chiropractic Examiners*, 744 S.W.2d 648, 657 (Tex. App. 1988); *Heinecke v. Department of Commerce*, 810 P.2d 459 (Utah App. 1991); *Pundy v. Department of Professional Regulation*, 570 N.E.2d 458 (Ill. App. 1991); *Perez v. Missouri State Board*, 803 S.W.2d 160 (Mo. App. 1991); *Haley v. Medical Disciplinary Board*, 818 P.2d 1062 (Wash. 1991).

19. 647 N.E.2d 996 (Ill. 1995).

20. See, e.g., Mo. Ann. Stat. § 334.100(2)(4)(i) (Vernon 1993); Nev. Rev. Stat. § 630.304(5) (1987).

21. See, e.g., Wyo. Stat. § 33-26-402(a)(vii) (1995).

22. For further analysis of the influence of the AMA Opinion on legal standards, see S. H. Johnson. 1993. "Judicial Review of Disciplinary Action for Sexual Misconduct in the Practice of Medicine." *Journal of the American Medical Association* 270 (13): 1586. Ethical standards of medical associations may be incorporated within licensure disciplinary standards by statute. See discussion in *Pons v. Ohio State Medical Board*, 614 N.E.2d 748 (Ohio 1993).

23. 818 P.2d 1062 (Wash. 1991).

24. See, e.g., Col. Rev. Stat. § 12-36-117(1)(r) (1995); and M. E. Norwood. 1995. "Changes in the Medical Practice Act." *Colorado Lawyer* 24: 2155.

25. 810 P.2d 459 (Utah App. 1991).

26. See also, *Ferguson v. People of State of Colorado*, 824 P.2d 803 (Colo. 1992); *In the Matter of Ackerman v. Ambach*, 142 AD2d 842, 530 N.Y.S.2d 893 (N.Y. App. 1988).

27. See, e.g., *Larocca v. State Board of Registration for the Healing Arts*, 897 S.W.2d 37 (Mo. App. 1995); *Andreski v. Commissioner of Education of State of New York*, 552 N.Y.S.2d 701 (N.Y. App. 1990). But see *In the Matter of H. Wang*, 441 N.W.2d 488 (Minn. 1989); *Lieberman v. Department of Professional Regulation*, 573 So.2d 349 (Fla. App. 1990).

28. See Chapter 5 below.

29. A. L. Hyams. 1993. "Expert Psychiatric Evidence in Sexual Misconduct Cases Before State Medical Boards." *American Journal of Law & Medicine* 18 (3): 171.

30. For a review of the literature documenting long-term adverse impact similar to rape or incest, post-traumatic stress disorder, and hospitalization, see Searight and Campbell, "Physician-Patient Sexual Contact," 247.

31. See review of the research in Council on Ethical and Judicial Affairs, "Sexual Misconduct."

32. "Ad Hoc Committee on Physician Impairment, Report on Sexual Boundary Issues." *Federation Bulletin* 82 (4): 208.

33. See further discussion in section on "Impairment" below.

34. See, e.g., *United States v. Jones*, 570 F.2d 765 (8th Cir. 1978); *United States v. Mahar*, 801 F.2d 1477 (6th Cir. 1986).

35. B. B. Wilford, J. Finch, D. J. Czechowicz, and D. Warren. 1994. "An Overview of Prescription Drug Misuse and Abuse: Defining the Problem and Seeking Solutions." *Journal of Law, Medicine & Ethics* 22 (3): 197; R. S. Shapiro. 1994. "Legal Bases for the Control of Analgesic Drugs." *Journal of Pain Symptom Management* 9 (April): 153.

36. See, e.g., K. L. Calderone. 1990. "The Influence of Gender and the Frequency of Pain and Sedative Medication Administered to Post-Operative Patients." *Sex Roles* 23: 713; K. H. Todd, N. Samaroo, and J. R. Hoffman. 1993. "Ethnicity as a Risk Factor for Inadequate Emergency Department Analgesia." *Journal of the American Medical Association* 269 (12): 1537.

37. Reported in F. J. Skelly. 1994. "Price of Pain Control: Is This the Risk You Face when Appropriately Prescribing Narcotics for Pain?" *American Medical News* 37 (16 May): 17.

38. F. J. Skelly. 1994. "Painful Barriers." *American Medical News* 37 (9 May): 15; Skelly, "Price of Pain Control," 17; F. J. Skelly. 1974. "Fear of Sanctions Limits Prescribing of Pain Drugs." *American Medical News* 37 (15 August): 19.

39. D. E. Joranson, C. S. Cleeland, D. E. Weissman, and A. M. Gilson. 1992. "Opioids for Chronic Cancer and Non-Cancer Pain: A Survey of State Medical Board Members." *Federation Bulletin* (June): 15–49.

40. D. E. Joranson. 1994. "Controlled Substances, Medical Practice and the Law." In *Psychiatric Practice under Fire: The Influence of Government, the Media, and Special Interests on Somatic Therapies*, edited by H. I. Schwartz. Washington, DC: American Psychiatric Press, Inc. 173–94.

41. See Chapter 2 above.

42. For one description of an investigation of suspected illegal prescriptive practices, see *Howard v. Miller*, 870 F.Supp. 340 (N.D. Ga. 1994). See also, R. N. Gaddis. 1993. "General Counsel Defends State Medical Licensure Board." *Journal of the Oklahoma State Medical Association* 86 (11): 561, responding to criticism of the board's handling of prescriptive practices cases.

43. 861 S.W.2d 317 (Ark. App. 1993).

44. *Hake v. Arkansas State Medical Board*, 374 S.W.2d 173 (Ark. 1964).

45. See *In the Matter of DiLeo*, 661 So.2d 162 (La. App. 1995), finding that duration of pain medication prescriptions "without proof that the prescriptions were rendered in an illegal or illegitimate manner" would not support disciplinary action based on breach of professional standards for prescription of controlled substances.

46. 1996 WL 346971 (Fla. App.).

47. See, e.g., *Fattah v. State Medical Board of Ohio*, 1994 WL 73903 (Ohio App. 1994); *Brown v. Louisiana State Board of Medical Examiners*, 637 So.2d 1113 (La. App. 1994); *In the Matter of DiLeo*, 661 So.2d 162 (La. App. 1995); *People v. Schade*, 32 Cal. Rptr. 2d 59 (Cal. App. 1994).

48. Consensus Statement, American Pain Society Quality of Care Committee. 1995. "Quality Improvement Guidelines for the Treatment of Acute Pain and Cancer Pain." *Journal of the American Medical Association* 274 (December): 1874; P. Crowley. 1994. "No Pain, No Gain?" The Agency for Health Care Policy and Research's Attempt to Change Inefficient Health Care Practice of Withholding Medication from Patients in Pain. *Journal of Contemporary Health Law and Policy* 10: 383; "*Acute Pain Management: Operative or Medical Procedures and Trauma*," Pub. No. 92-0021, Agency for Health Care Policy and Research (Feb. 1992); *Management of Cancer Pain: Clinical Practice Guidelines*, Pub. No. 94-0592, Agency for Health Care Policy and Research (March 1994).

49. See, e.g., *Hoover v. Agency for Health Care Administration*, 1996 WL 346971 (Fla. App.).

50. 661 So.2d 162 (La. App. 1995).

51. 32 Cal. Rptr. 2d 59 (Cal. App. 1994).

52. D. E. Joranson and A. M. Gilson. 1994. "Policy Issues and Imperatives in the Use of Opioids to Treat Pain in Substance Abusers." *Journal of Law, Medicine & Ethics* 22 (Fall): 215.

53. S. R. Savage. 1993. "Pain Medicine and Addiction Medicine—Controversies and Collaboration." *Journal of Pain Symptom Management* 8 (5): 254.

54. But see *Reynolds v. Louisiana State Board of Medical Examiners*, 646 So.2d 1244 (La. App. 1994), holding that boards' discipline of physician for prescription of controlled substances for persons who were "abusing" was supported by sufficient evidence.

55. Quoting *People v. Victor*, 62 Cal. 2d 280, 42 Cal. Rptr. 199, 398 P.2d 391 (Cal. 1965).

56. D. E. Joranson. 1995. "State Medical Board Guidelines for Treatment of Intractable Pain," *American Pain Society Bulletin* (May/June): 1.

57. State of California, Summit on Effective Pain Management: Removing Impediments to Appropriate Prescribing (March 18, 1994); Medical Board of California, Statement by the Medical Board and Action Report (July 1994).

58. Cal. Bus. & Prof. Code § 2241.5 (West 1994); Fla. Stat. Ann. § 458.326 (West 1995); Mo. Ann. Stat. § 334.105 et seq. (Vernon 1995); Nev. Rev. Stat. § 630.3066 (1995); N.D. Cent. Code § 19-03.3-01 et seq. (1995); Or. Rev. Stat. § 677.470 et seq. (1995); Tex. Rev. Civ. Stat. Ann. art. 4495c (West 1996); Va. Code Ann. § 54.1-3408.1 (Michie 1995).

59. See generally, D. E. Joranson. 1996. "Intractable Pain Treatment Laws and Regulations." *American Pain Society Bulletin* 24 (4): 1.

60. See, e.g., Mo. Ann. Stat. § 334.105(2)(3) (Vernon 1995).

61. See Chapter 4 below.

62. D. J. Behr. 1994. "Prescription Drug Control Under the Federal Controlled Substances Act: A Web of Administrative, Civil, and Criminal Law Controls." *Washington University Journal of Urban and Contemporary Law* 45 (Winter): 41. See, e.g., *Smith v. California State Board of Pharmacy*, 37 Cal. App. 4th 229, 43 Cal. Rptr. 2d 532 (Cal. App. 1995).

63. Prescription monitoring systems have a substantial effect on access to treatment for pain. J. H. VonRoenn, C. S. Cleeland, R. Gonin, A. K. Hatfield, and K. J. Pandya. 1993. "Physician Attitudes and Practice in Cancer Pain Management: A Survey from the Eastern Cooperative Oncology Group." *Annotated Internal Medicine* 119 (2): 121.

64. See, e.g., Cal. Bus. & Prof. Code § 2241.5(e) (West 1994).

65. Fla. Stat. Ann. § 458.326 (West 1995); Nev. Rev. Stat. § 630.3066 (1995).

66. Or. Rev. Stat. § 677.485 (1995).

67. N.D. Cent. Code § 19-13.3-03 (1995); Tex. Rev. Civ. Stat. Ann, art. 4495c(4) (West 1996).

68. Federation of State Medical Boards, Survey of State Medical Boards, in Report of the Ad Hoc Committee on Physician Impairment (Appendix) (April 1995). See also West's Ann. Cal. Bus. & Prof. Code § 2770 (impaired nurse program); Colo. Rev. St. Ann. § 12-38-131 (for all health professionals).

69. 1995. Ad Hoc Committee on Physician Impairment, "Report on Sexual Boundary

Issues." *Federation Bulletin* 82 (4): 208.

70. P. Hughes, N. Brandenburg, D. C. Balwin, Jr., C. L. Storr, and K. M. Williams. 1992. "Prevalence of Substance Abuse among U.S. Physicians." *Journal of the American Medical Association* 267 (6 May): 2333.

71. W. E. McAuliffe, N. Rohman, S. Santangelo, E. Magnuson, D. Anthony, D. V. Sheehan, A. Sobol, and J. Weissman. 1986. "Psychoactive Drug Use among Practicing Physicians and Medical Students." *New England Journal of Medicine* 315 (13): 805.

72. J. L. Anderson. 1994. "Treatment Considerations for the Addicted Nurse." *Behavioral Health Management* 14 (5): 22; H. Lippmann and S. Nagle. 1992. "Addicted Nurses: Tolerated, Tormented, or Treated?" *RN* 55: 55.

73. See, e.g., W. E. McAuliffe, N. Rohman, P. Breer, G. Wynshak, S. Santangelo, E. Magnuson, R. D. Moore, L. Mead, and T. A. Pearson. 1991. "Alcohol Use and Abuse in Random Samples of Physicians and Medical Students." *American Journal of Public Health* 81 (2): 177, comparing physicians to lawyers; R. D. Moore, L. Mead, and T. A. Pearson. "Youthful Precursors of Alcohol Abuse in Physicians." *American Journal of Medicine* 88 (4): 332.

74. R. D. Moore, L. Mead, and T. A. Pearson. 1990. "Youthful Precursors of Alcohol Abuse in Physicians." *American Journal of Medicine* 88 (4): 332.

75. K. Gallegos and J. Kelly. 1990. "Trends in Physician Drug Abuse: Prevention and Control." *Addiction & Recovery* 10: 28; K. L. Sprinkle. 1994. "Physician Alcoholism: A Survey of the Literature." *Federation Bulletin* 81 (2): 113.

76. See, e.g., Cal. Bus. & Prof. Code § 2762 (West 1984); 225 ILCS 65/25(b)(9) (1993); N.Y. Educ. Law § 6509(3) (McKinney 1980).

77. P. Hughes et al., "Prevalence of Substance Abuse."

78. See, e.g., C. Winick. 1991. "Social Behavior, Public Policy, and Nonharmful Drug Use." *Milbank Quarterly* 69 (3): 437, arguing that the use of drugs in and of itself should not be presumed to be conclusive evidence of impairment as regular users of heroin, cocaine, and other psychoactive drugs are often able to function effectively at work.

79. See, e.g., 225 ILCS 65/25(b)(9) (1993).

80. See, e.g., Cal. Bus. & Prof. Code § 2762 (1984).

81. See, e.g., *O'Brien v. Commission of Education of State of New York*, 523 N.Y.S.2d 680 (N.Y. App. 1988).

82. See, e.g., *Arkansas State Medical Board v. Young*, 1994 WL 494622 (Ark. App. 1994), reversing sanction against licensee and holding that a doctor's suicide attempt does not indicate that the doctor's continuation in practice endangers the public.

83. See, e.g., Miss. Code Ann. § 73-15-29(1)(h) (1991).

84. See also, concerning the definition of alcoholism, K. L. Sprinkle. 1994. "Physician Alcoholism: A Survey of the Literature." *Federation Bulletin* 81 (2): 113.

85. 624 So.2d 485 (Miss. 1993).

86. See also *Colorado State Board of Nursing v. Lang*, 842 P.2d 1383 (Colo. App. 1992).

87. 495 N.W.2d 698 (Iowa 1993).

88. See, e.g., *Corder v. Kansas Board of Healing Arts*, 889 P.2d 1127 (Kan. 1994); *Lepley v. Department of Health*, 190 A.D.2d 556, 593 N.Y.S.2d 235 (N.Y. App. 1993).

89. See, e.g., *Humenansky v. Minnesota Board of Medical Examiners*, 525 N.W.2d 559 (Minn. App. 1994); *Kees v. Medical Board of California*, 7 Cal. App. 4th 1801, 10 Cal. Rptr. 2d 112 (Cal. App. 1992).

90. Federation of State Medical Boards, Survey of State Medical Boards, in Report of the Ad Hoc Committee on Physician Impairment (Appendix) (April 1995).

91. See, e.g., C. Morrow. 1984. "Doctors Helping Doctors." *Hastings Center Report* 14 (6): 32.

92. Lippman and Nagle. 1992. "Addicted Nurses: Tolerated, Tormented, or Treated?" 36.

93. See *Federation Bulletin* 82 (3): 125, for articles describing programs in several states. See also, J. L. Anderson. 1994. "Treatment Considerations for the Addicted Nurse." *Behavioral Health Management* 14 (Sept.–Oct.): 22.

94. R. Walzer. 1990. "Impaired Physicians: An Overview and Update of the Legal Issues." *Journal of Legal Medicine* 11 (2): 131.

95. Federation of State Medical Boards, Report of the Ad Hoc Committee on Physician Impairment, April 1995.

96. C. Morrow. 1984. "Doctors Helping Doctors." *Hastings Center Report* 14 (6): 32.

97. 7 Cal. App. 4th 1801, 10 Cal. Rptr. 2d 112 (Cal. App. 1992).

98. M. F. Fleming. 1994. "Physician Impairment: Options for Intervention." *American Family Physician* 50 (July): 41.

99. B. Schneidman. 1995. "Editorial: The Philosophy of Rehabilitation for Impaired Physicians." *Federation Bulletin* 82 (3): 125.

100. Sprinkle, "Physician Alcoholism."

101. 42 U.S.C. § 12101 et seq. (1990).

102. 42 U.S.C. § 12102(2) (1990).

103. 28 C.F.R. § 35.130(b)(6) (1991).

104. Medical licensure boards are also subject to the Act in their functions as employer and as public entities offering services under Titles I and III of the Act.

105. The Act provides that state agencies do not have immunity from damages claims under the Act. 42 U.S.C. § 12202 (1990). But see *Seminole Tribe of Florida v. Florida*, 116 S.Ct. 1114 (1996), for a recent and restrictive analysis of constitutional restrictions on Congress's authority to limit Eleventh Amendment immunity.

106. 42 U.S.C. § 12102(2) (1990).

107. 42 U.S.C. § 12114 (1990).

108. 28 C.F.R. § 35.131(a) and (b) (1991).

109. See discussion of *Mississippi State Board of Nursing v. Wilson*, supra.

110. *Colorado State Board of Medical Examiners v. Davis*, 893 P.2d 1365 (Colo. App. 1995).

111. *Southeastern Community College v. Davis*, 442 U.S. 397 (1979).

112. See, e.g., *In re Rubenstein*, 637 A.2d 1131 (Del. 1994).

113. 28 C.F.R. Pt. 35, App. A. (1991).

114. 480 U.S. 273 (1987).

115. 921 F.Supp. 482 (W.D.Mich. 1995).

116. See also, *Ramachandar v. Sobol*, 838 F.Supp. 100 (S.D.N.Y. 1993), holding that

board decision on issue of accommodation was entitled to some deference in claim under the Rehabilitation Act.

117. 1993 WL 413016 (D.N.J.).

118. See, e.g., *Alexander v. Margolis*, 921 F.Supp. 482 (W.D.Mich. 1995); *Florida Bar v. Clement*, 662 So.2d 690 (Fla. 1995).

REGULATING INTERDISCIPLINARY PRACTICE

William M. Sage and Linda H. Aiken

THE LANGUAGE of doctors and nurses has undergone subtle but significant shifts over the past two decades. The word "medicine," for example, has largely been replaced by the more inclusive "healthcare," and "physician" now frequently gives way to the more diverse "health professional." With one exception, however, economic clout and political power have not kept pace with semantic progress.

The exception is the phrase "healthcare industry." Previously describing pharmaceutical manufacturers and insurance companies, current usage encompasses new modes of healthcare delivery such as managed care, and includes professional and charitable domains as well as clearly corporate ones. Today's healthcare industry—accounting for nearly one trillion dollars in annual spending[1]—is redefining professional roles and responsibilities that have been well established since the early years of the century.

For individuals who provide healthcare services, current market instability carries with it both risks and opportunities: risks of losing hard-won professional privileges, and opportunities to expand authority over contested, unclaimed, or uncharted practice territories. For legislators and policymakers, today's market brings three major challenges: how to monitor the business contracts that are redefining professional relationships in healthcare; how to enforce the social contracts that set healthcare apart from other commercial pursuits; and how to govern during a period of rapid change.

This chapter considers the law and other publicly sanctioned practices that affect health professionals other than physicians. These professionals fall roughly into three groups, according to the manner in which patients obtain their services. Some, such as advanced practice nurses and physician assistants, act as initial contacts for individuals seeking general healthcare.[2] Others, such as chiropractors, psychologists, and podiatrists, provide specialized services to patients referred by primary care providers or, in some cases, who seek their services on a self-referred basis.[3] Still others, such as registered nurses and various allied health professionals, serve predominantly in assistive roles to primary care providers and specialists.[4]

The chapter concludes that, in today's more sophisticated, corporatized healthcare system, debates traditionally framed in terms of interprofessional boundaries should be recast in terms of interprofessional relationships. Regulatory efforts increasingly should be focused on institutional structures and processes, and on informing as well as protecting consumers. Because the determinants of these interprofessional relationships are complex and changeable, however, legal standards alone are unlikely to achieve public policy goals with respect to the health professions.

Overview of Interdisciplinary Regulation

Following World War II, scientific advances transformed healthcare from a cottage industry to a sophisticated enterprise requiring both specialization and coordination.[5] Demand evolved as well, with employers and government becoming dominant purchasers. Resource constraints gradually led to price-consciousness, competition, and accelerating integration and consolidation of care in larger organizations. Bioethical insights, the consumer protection movement, and the information revolution contributed to the decline of medical paternalism and encouraged new approaches to health and disease. Finally, the repeated failure to enact national health insurance allowed the healthcare industry to develop piecemeal in each state, while leaving large sections of the population uninsured and therefore at risk.

Like the multicentric healthcare system to which they relate, the laws and regulations governing the health professions are complex.[6] Some laws explicitly set forth the rights and privileges of health professionals, while others exert indirect but significant effects on professional relationships. In addition, private, governmentally sanctioned activities often determine practice opportunities.

Federal and state laws that govern the healthcare professions include the following:

- state licensure, certification, and registration laws establishing scope of practice;
- unauthorized practice statutes enforced by professional discipline or criminal penalties;
- laws determining the structure and control of professional disciplinary authority;
- federal food and drug laws limiting treatments to prescription use;
- judicial interpretations of "medical necessity" and other provisions in health insurance contracts;
- mandated benefit laws (subject to ERISA preemption);
- open-panel legislation such as "any-willing-provider" and "freedom-of-choice" laws (again, subject to ERISA preemption);
- Medicare participation and reimbursement provisions;
- Medicaid participation and reimbursement provisions;
- workers' compensation participation and reimbursement provisions;
- credentialing procedures and medical staff governance;
- private accreditation and certification standards given force of law;
- labor and employment laws;
- corporate practice prohibitions and professional corporation laws;
- antitrust statutes and government enforcement policies;
- professional liability laws and judicial decisions;
- financial responsibility and liability insurance laws; and
- health education funding laws.

In the next section, we describe the major sources of interdisciplinary regulation—legal licensure, institutional affiliations, insurance reimbursement, and financing of professional education—which matured in the fee-for-service health system that characterized American medicine's post-war expansion. The section that follows relates these regulatory processes to the principal forces at work during the transformation to managed care after 1980—consolidation and cost-containment—and identifies broader issues of individual rights and social responsibility that are likely to prove important to the future of interdisciplinary practice.

The Fee-for-Service Paradigm: Autonomy and Protectionism

Although its roots go back over two hundred years, professional regulation took its modern form between 1950 and 1980. This period was characterized by one mode of healthcare delivery, fee-for-service practice, and one mode of healthcare financing, cost-based (or charge-based) third-party payment. Under third-party payment, increasing the availability of services induced additional consumption rather than decreasing price, confounding classical notions of supply and demand. As a result, competition during this time—if it can be called competition at all—was more often between classes of providers than between individuals. Public acceptance and therefore access to insurance reimbursement were the keys to clinical autonomy and financial success, with each health profession fighting to secure some portion of the privilege that society accorded physicians.

Licensure

In healthcare as in other regulated industries, the economic interests of regulated entities motivate a considerable portion of regulatory activity. Professional licensing laws are a prime example. All fifty states require healthcare professionals to possess valid licenses or certificates based on education, examination, and supervised practice experience.[7] Licensure qualifies the recipient to provide healthcare services to the public within the scope of practice established by the relevant "professional practice act" in each state, subject to oversight by the appropriate professional disciplinary body. Although justified in terms of public safety, mandatory professional licensure also confers economic advantage on individuals who meet legally specified qualifications, limiting consumer choices and producer responses while increasing costs.[8]

Practice acts for physicians are usually all-encompassing, and are enforced against infringing practitioners by equally broad state criminal laws prohibiting the "unauthorized practice of medicine."[9] Medicine is noteworthy among modern professions for having staked out far more territory than physicians themselves can service, and for managing that territory by delegating duties to other professions who remain subject to physician control and supervision. In part because the cost of care has been, until recently, a secondary consideration, direct challenges to physician supremacy were usually rebuffed on quality grounds. As a result, the majority of other licensed health professionals—even those with rich professional traditions of their own, such as midwives—have been forced to define or redefine themselves with reference to a physician-directed healthcare system.[10]

Organized medicine has consistently opposed efforts to place specialty-based limits on medical licenses. Consequently, the actual scope of physician practice is determined largely by nongovernmental factors such as availability of training, and access to hospital privileges, network affiliations, and malpractice insurance. By contrast, practice acts for other health professionals typically identify a specific range of permitted services and attach conditions to delivering them. For example, 48 states and the District of Columbia currently regulate advanced practice nurses.[11] Typical practice restrictions include requiring supervision by a licensed physician (15 states), mandating compliance with written protocols (35 states), and withholding the right to prescribe medication independently (38 states).[12] In a few states, location (e.g., rural areas or community health clinics) is a further condition limiting advanced nursing practice. Physician assistants practice under similar terms and conditions.[13]

Health professionals such as dentists, chiropractors, and optometrists are generally authorized to treat patients without physician supervision or referral, but are limited in their licensed scope of practice. In California, for example, chiropractors may treat almost all medical conditions, and may order, perform, and interpret diagnostic tests, but may not prescribe medications, practice surgery, or care for obstetrical patients.[14]

Favored professions have often used licensing criteria to retain control over the delivery of healthcare services and related revenues.[15] Struggles between physicians and midwives over maternity services date back several hundred years, and still continue in many parts of the world.[16] Similarly, psychologists have sought parity in some areas with psychiatrists, optometrists have coveted procedures performed by ophthalmologists, and dental hygienists have challenged some practices of dentists.[17] During the 1993–94 health reform debate, proposals that nurse practitioners serve as low-cost "family doctors" prompted an aggressive campaign by organized medicine deriding independent nurse practice as quackery. Organized nursing bridled at these charges, while simultaneously decrying the performance of nursing tasks by cheaper, unlicensed assistive personnel using similarly broad, quality-based rhetoric.[18]

Although practice acts for nonphysician professionals generally provide that compliance with their terms does not constitute the unauthorized practice of medicine, the supposedly exclusive scope of licensed medical practice frequently leads to litigation, given statutory ambiguities and overlapping competencies.[19] Similarly, assignment of tasks to nonprofessional personnel may land healthcare providers in court.[20]

Even members of what is nominally the same occupation may sue one another; for example, associations of *registered* nurses have challenged the extension of additional hospital duties to licensed vocational or practical nurses.[21] Litigation of this sort serves as a reminder that calls for certification of currently unlicensed workers may backfire by giving rise to yet another formally recognized, and competitive, category of health professional.

Recent instability in the healthcare system has intensified conflicts over scope of practice, leading to a spate of legislative reforms. Approximately 400 bills were introduced in state legislatures in 1994, and 135 laws enacted, to expand the scope of practice of various health professionals.[22] Some states have even undertaken more comprehensive evaluations of their regulatory schemes for the health professions.[23]

For example, the right to prescribe medication is hotly contested.[24] Most states now grant physician assistants and advanced practice nurses some degree of prescriptive authority.[25] These professionals write nearly one million prescriptions each month nationwide, double the number written four years ago, but still barely more than one-half of one percent of all medication prescribed.[26] In recognition of recent changes in state law, the federal Drug Enforcement Agency (DEA) began issuing permits for controlled substances to advanced practice nurses and physician assistants in 1995.

Interest group politics can confound public policy considerations where licensure laws are concerned. For example, a broad coalition of providers and consumers in New York was able to secure the passage in 1992 of a practice act for professional midwifery in order to expand access to services and promote consumer choice.[27] To their consternation, the statute was almost immediately invoked by newly licensed professionals to reduce competition from established practitioners who did not meet the nursing education requirements of the new law but who had been tolerated under the prior, more general enforcement scheme.[28]

Recognizing these problems, the Institute of Medicine recommended in a 1996 report that state governments review scope-of-practice laws for primary care nurse practitioners and physician assistants, and eliminate or modify restrictions that impede collaborative practice and reduce access to care.[29] The Pew Health Professions Commission has also advocated sweeping changes to state professional practice acts and enforcement, including standardized language, entry requirements based solely on competence assessments, overlapping scopes of practice, and interdisciplinary, publicly accountable oversight boards.[30] Noting that "[d]espite one profession's demonstration of competence . . . [it] must also engage in political battles with other professions," the Pew Commission urged the elimination of exclusive professional domains—and thereby litigation over what constitutes "unauthorized practice" of a rival profession.[31]

A more systematic approach is to identify tasks that present demonstrable risks to the public, and constrain them to licensed health professionals. For example, an innovative regulatory system now in effect in Ontario specifies thirteen "controlled acts" that are considered potentially hazardous, while companion laws authorize each of the province's 24 licensed professions to perform none, some, or all of those acts.[32] Tasks not falling within these areas, even if traditionally associated with the health professions, may be performed by unlicensed personnel.

Supervision Requirements

The issue of physician "supervision" as a legal condition of practice for other health professionals merits separate attention. The creation of a clinical hierarchy serves several purposes, ranging from economic dominance to accountability for error. A prominent feature of licensure laws for advanced practice nurses, physician assistants, and certain other health professionals, supervision requirements are also found in reimbursement contracts and statutes, medical staff procedures, and professional liability policies.

Whether particular professionals accept a subordinate role to physicians often depends on their history and traditions. For example, nursing is based on fundamentally different conceptions of health and professional service than medicine is. As a result, advanced practice nurses are trained as autonomous professionals, and neither aspire to replace physicians nor rely on them for constant assistance with clinical decision making. By contrast, physician assistants are trained in medical settings to work under physician tutelage. They therefore view themselves—and are treated by the law—as agents of their supervising physicians.[33]

As might be expected, the content of laws establishing clinical hierarchies and the terminology used—such as "supervision," "collaboration," or "joint practice"—are heavily negotiated. The effects of these provisions vary widely. Many are largely ignored in practice, while others merely increase costs to patients through higher overhead or explicit billing of supervisory services to payors. Some supervision requirements, however, significantly chill interdisciplinary practice because medical societies, hospital medical staffs, or physician-controlled malpractice insurers successfully discourage physicians from serving in their legally mandated capacities. For example, nurse-midwives who are legally required to have a collaboration agreement in place have sometimes been unable to find obstetricians who would agree to treat their patients if medical intervention became necessary.[34]

Like other laws and regulations originally intended to protect physician hegemony, supervision requirements have trickled down the economic ladder, to be invoked by various professions against newcomers. In the face of hospitals' increased use of minimally trained workers to perform traditional nursing duties, for example, organized nursing has echoed organized medicine's defensive posture by requiring tasks to be "delegated by and under the supervision of the registered professional nurse,"[35] and several state boards of nursing have issued regulations and advisory opinions with respect to unlicensed personnel.[36]

Professional Discipline

At least as important as the specified scope of practice in each state is the administrative structure for disciplining health professionals. Only with effort have licensed professionals other than physicians secured the right to police their own members. In eight states, the board of *medicine* still has some authority over advanced practice nurses.[37] Overlapping or ambiguous jurisdiction by professional boards predisposes to litigation.[38] Even where each profession has its own disciplinary structure, the legislative prohibition on unauthorized medical practice often permits the medical board to challenge activities of nonphysician practitioners and other professional boards.

The Pew Health Professions Commission has noted the conflict of interest inherent in vesting professional self-regulatory boards with governmental authority. The Pew Commission therefore suggested the creation of an interdisciplinary oversight board to coordinate health professions regulation in each state, the restructuring of individual professional boards based on practice overlap, and the expansion of public representation.[39] Virginia has maintained such a "superboard" since 1977.[40] Called the Board of Health Professions, it comprises one member from each of Virginia's twelve individual professional boards plus five citizen members. The Pew Commission also urged the establishment of uniform complaint and disciplinary processes to identify and prosecute incompetent practitioners.[41]

In any case, the degree to which legal restrictions are honored remains uncertain. As with many public enforcement schemes, resource constraints and the large number of regulated professionals and transactions make effective oversight difficult. Anecdotal evidence suggests that considerable unlicensed practice occurs, as does practice outside the authorized scope of a health professional license. For example, requirements that physicians supervise advanced practice nurses and physician assistants are rarely followed. Similarly, more than half of nurse practitioners in states that do not grant prescriptive authority nonetheless prescribe medications for common ailments.[42]

Institutional Affiliations

The modern hospital has been largely responsible for the social pre-eminence and economic prosperity of the medical profession. Institutional affiliations are also prerequisites to successful practice for many nonphysician health professionals. For example, nurse practitioners and clinical psychologists may require hospital admitting privileges to provide inpatient care to a subset of their patients. Similarly, nurse-midwives depend on support and referral relationships should complications arise during labor and delivery. Without these resources, many such practitioners have little choice but to become employees of physicians or hospitals.

Several features of hospitals have allowed physicians to assert control over the practices of other health professionals. These include hospitals' general financial dependence on physicians for referrals, the organization of nursing and ancillary care into service-based rather than patient-based departments, and the right of self-governing medical staffs to decide who may treat patients in the hospital.

Hospitals (and, increasingly, potential contract partners such as managed care companies) also typically require affiliated professionals to be covered by malpractice insurance. Similarly, some state regulators require licensed professionals who see patients "independently" to be adequately insured.[43] Liability insurance may be difficult to obtain for many nonphysician practitioners, further encouraging them to become employees of insured practitioners or institutions. Approximately half of the individual malpractice coverage in the United States is underwritten by physician-owned mutuals. Many of these companies do not insure health professionals other than physicians, or are accessed only through membership in local medical societies. In addition, physician-dominated insurers have sometimes imposed hefty surcharges not commensurate with risk on physicians who collaborate with other health professionals.[44] Because of these market distortions, most American nurse-midwives lost their malpractice insurance in 1985 when their primary commercial carrier declined to renew coverage.[45]

Federal antitrust remedies are available in some cases, although litigation is time-consuming and expensive. In one instance, a chiropractor successfully sued the AMA under a boycott theory for engaging in a concerted campaign to prevent clinical collaboration or joint teaching or research.[46] Physician-controlled Blue Shield plans have also been vulnerable to antitrust challenges.[47] On the other hand, courts tend to approve conduct by hospitals (or other entities not controlled by physicians) that has procompetitive effects, even though certain provider groups are excluded.[48]

Third-Party Payment

Either openly or tacitly, the majority of legal and political disputes among healthcare professionals have focused on access to the "golden goose" of insurance reimbursement. A right to reimbursement means a secure source of income, not only supporting operating expenses but allowing health professionals to borrow additional capital to establish or expand their practices. As a result, battles among health professions, and between professionals and payors, are frequently fought in state legislatures or the Federal Congress over mandated benefits, workers' compensation coverage, and the terms of Medicare and Medicaid reimbursement.

Private Insurance

Private insurance practices reinforce the physician orientation of health-care. For example, standard indemnity insurance policies cover treatment within defined benefit categories (e.g., hospital services or laboratory services) that is "medically necessary," often defined as care ordered by a physician, not solely for convenience and in accordance with generally accepted medical practice.[49] Courts have frequently interpreted these clauses in a manner deferential to the medical profession, creating a presumption in favor of necessity if supported by the patient's "treating physician," a standard that continues to govern cases relating to Medicare benefits.[50]

State legislatures and insurance regulators have imposed additional coverage requirements on private insurers in response to lobbying by nonphysician health professionals and their patients. Legislation frequently takes the form of nondiscrimination provisions. Approximately half of the states require direct reimbursement to chiropractors if coverage includes any services within their scope of practice, and several states extend similar privileges to providers such as clinical psychologists, social workers, podiatrists, and acupuncturists.[51] In a few states, laws have been proposed or enacted expressly mandating coverage of specific services such as chiropractic.[52]

States may also enact open-panel legislation. Any-willing-provider laws require insurers to contract with, and therefore reimburse, the services of any provider willing to meet their basic terms and conditions. Freedom-of-choice laws allow insured individuals to obtain care from any licensed professional and to claim reimbursement regardless of the existence of a contract between the professional and the plan. Although these laws are now being backed by physicians concerned about managed care, they traditionally protected politically powerful groups of nonphysician professionals such as independent pharmacists, podiatrists, and chiropractors.

The major legal impediment to both mandated-benefit and open-panel laws is the federal Employee Retirement Income Security Act of 1974 (ERISA),[53] which preempts many state efforts to regulate the payment practices of employer-sponsored health plans. For example, states may not enforce mandated-benefit and any-willing-provider laws against the growing number of employers who self-insure.[54] Although laws regulating insurance are not preempted, courts are divided as to whether contracts between insurers and providers, as opposed to policyholders, constitute the business of insurance.[55]

Government Health Programs

Medicare and Medicaid conditions of participation and reimbursement requirements are perhaps the most important laws affecting practice structure and interprofessional relationships.[56] Like private insurers, Medicare and Medicaid cover only services within specified categories, generally linked to the professional license of the provider. Because these two programs account for about 40 percent of healthcare spending, their requirements constitute de facto practice acts for many health professionals.[57]

Nonphysician health professionals have lobbied successfully for Medicare reimbursement. The statute's definition of "physician" now includes dentists, podiatrists, optometrists, and chiropractors.[58] Other provisions mandate coverage of the services of psychologists, many advanced practice nurses, and selected allied health practitioners.[59]

However, nonphysician practitioners may not receive equal pay for equal work, may be required to bill for their services through a physician, and may be limited to practice in parts of the country with recognized shortages of health professionals. For example, Medicare permits nurse practitioners and physician assistants to receive direct reimbursement only in rural areas, and only at 75 to 85 percent of physician payment levels.[60] Nurse practitioners must collaborate with, and physician assistants must be supervised by (and billed through), a physician. In other areas (except for nursing home settings, where special rules apply), the services of advanced practice nurses are only eligible for Medicare payment if delivered "incident to" physician services and provided under supervision; these are billed by the physician at the physician's rate.

Federal Medicaid law requires states to cover the services of certified family nurse practitioners, certified pediatric nurse practitioners, and certified nurse-midwives.[61] Services of optometrists and chiropractors receive federal funding if states elect to cover them.[62] Several states have also extended non–federally matched coverage to other advanced practice nurses and other health professionals.[63]

Legislatures facing budget constraints are often reluctant to fund services by new groups of health professionals, and courts have generally upheld their decisions.[64] For government programs structured on a fee-for-service rather than prepaid basis, allowing direct reimbursement of nonphysician health professionals is a financial gamble—overall expenditures might increase even though each service is delivered at lower cost.[65] These considerations should not apply to Medicare and Medicaid managed care programs where the only government payment is an annual premium.

Professional Education

The structure and financing of professional education have been among the most important legal determinants of professional relations and practice opportunities. The makeup of the U.S. healthcare work force is neither serendipitous nor market driven. Rather, it reflects a series of legislative decisions, some motivated by public policy and others by political expediency, to channel public investment in particular directions. These decisions sometimes create ambiguous incentives for cost and quality, and result in markets for professional training that are seldom contiguous with the markets governing practice.

Of the health professions, only medicine has been able to control both general training and specialty opportunities. By contrast, educational programs for nursing and allied health vary widely in admission requirements, classroom and clinical curricula, location of training, tuition, financial support, and credential awarded. For example, there are three pathways leading to registered nurse licensure: three-year hospital diploma programs, two-year associate degree programs offered at junior or community colleges, and baccalaureate programs in four-year colleges and universities.

Heterogeneity of practice preparation poses a dilemma with respect to work force supply. On the one hand, it increases individual opportunity for entry into these professions. On the other, it weakens intraprofessional cohesiveness, hampering the ability of graduates to define themselves to other professions, governing bodies, and the public at large. As a result, many professions and the institutions that train them compete fiercely for limited resources, or are wholly unable to attract public investment in education.

Only physicians receive government funding for graduate education (over $2 billion annually in direct payments alone) on a per-trainee basis.[66] Subsidies for other health professionals, if they exist at all, are generally aggregate payments that are not controlled by the nominal beneficiaries and therefore correlate poorly with actual training. For example, federal Graduate Nurse Education (GNE) funding goes entirely to hospital-based diploma nurse programs whose graduates are already in oversupply and who are frequently unqualified for advanced nursing education.[67] Even federal payments for physician education are linked to Medicare hospital reimbursement formulas. This has contributed to a surplus of expensively trained medical specialists, while shortchanging health professions that provide only outpatient services.

Financing of professional education might profitably be restructured to expand the diversity of practice settings, promote interdisciplinary training, and provide per-trainee support of all health professionals who are qualified to deliver primary care services. It is noteworthy that the length of training for American advanced practice nurses is roughly comparable to that of generalist physician education in most industrialized nations. Moreover, collaborative practice requires cooperative, collegial relationships that are best established through commonalities of training and professional socialization.

Federalism and Interprofessional Regulation

The foregoing sections demonstrate the uniquely American division of regulatory authority over healthcare between federal and state governments. For example, licensure of occupations is generally a state prerogative, although the importance of Medicare and Medicaid reimbursement policies to the viability of practice creates a substantial federal presence.[68] An important question is whether a more direct national role in the regulation of health professionals is warranted. Proposals have been made to supersede state laws defining scope of practice with federal legislation. The Clinton Administration's Health Security Act, for example, would have preempted any state law that restricted health professionals "beyond what is justified by [their] skills and training."[69]

Uniformity is possible without federal intervention. The Pew Commission favors consistent regulatory terminology and uniform standards for entry to practice which directly measure knowledge and skills, with interstate reciprocal licensure by endorsement.[70] The Physician Payment Review Commission similarly endorsed the development of model practice acts for nonphysician practitioners.[71] The Council on Licensure, Enforcement, and Regulation, the National Governors' Association, the National Conference of State Legislatures, and other national associations of professional regulatory boards have proposed regulatory models using standardized terminology. Montana recently became the first state to adopt a Uniform Licensing Act for all professional and technical occupations.[72]

Arguments can be made for federal legislation. Inconsistent state laws may make it difficult for many health professionals to relocate to another state. Unlike professions such as law, where knowledge is state specific, training in the health professions is science based and universal. State laws also constitute a barrier to cost-effective, collaborative methods of services such as telemedicine, because health professionals rendering care by electronic means must nonetheless be licensed in the state in which the patient is located.[73] In addition, as demonstrated by the events leading to the creation of the National Practitioner Data Bank, lack of regulatory coordination may result in substandard professionals being admitted to practice when providers relocate.

However, arguments to federalize professional practice may also represent an attempt by groups disenfranchised in state legislatures to reverse their defeats through congressional action. As Briffault has observed, one consequence of a federal system is that battles lost in one forum can be refought in another.[74] An obvious example is medical malpractice reform, which bounces between state legislatures, state constitutional courts, and the federal Congress.

The Managed Care Paradigm: Integration and Interdependency

In business as in evolution, environmental change rewards diversity. Throughout history, professions have enlarged their spheres of influence, and new professions have arisen, in response to outside forces.[75] This is confirmed by the recent history of healthcare, where market competition and corporatization have altered many of the assumptions on which professional traditions and regulatory responses were based. Vertical integration of insurance financing with delivery of services and horizontal integration of small providers into large organizations are the hallmarks of today's healthcare system. Despite inevitable dislocations, this more disciplined healthcare economy creates opportunities for innovation and cooperation that were lacking in the era of physician dominance and cost-insensitive third-party payment.

Consolidation and Cost Containment

In the absence of meaningful cost constraints, competition between professions was conducted largely in the political arena.[76] Now, competition occurs primarily in the marketplace, involving firms and entrepreneurs as well as interest groups. As a result, decisions to substitute one class of health professional for another, or conversely to use their skills in a complementary manner, are increasingly being made through decentralized market processes, rather than through aggregate political judgments.

Hospitals

The introduction of Medicare prospective payment for hospitals in 1983 signaled a new era in which extended inpatient stays generated costs rather than revenues, beginning a cycle of hospital downsizing that continues today. Managed care accelerated this process, taking advantage of excess bed capacity and high fixed costs to negotiate steep discounts. Length of stay decreased, hospital occupancy dropped further, marginal facilities merged or closed, and severity of illness rose.

Surviving hospitals have witnessed significant changes in employment.[77] The number of registered nurses—capable of caring for the current generation of sicker, more complicated inpatients—has actually increased.[78] However, overall nurse staffing has decreased, particularly employment of vocational or practical nurses, many of whose duties have been assumed by unlicensed workers.

Hospitals have also experimented with other ways of reducing costs, including using physician assistants and advanced practice nurses to substitute for hospital-based physicians.[79] For example, nurse anesthetists are able to perform routine clinical tasks with minimal supervision.[80] Similarly, cutbacks in funding for academic health centers have led to the hiring of advanced practice nurses to assume duties traditionally delegated to interns and residents.[81]

As might be expected, hospital bed reductions, mergers, and closures have provoked employee unrest, particularly among unionized nurses.[82] In response, hospitals have challenged unions' legitimacy and right to bargain.[83] Nursing groups alleging diminished quality of care have also taken their cases to state legislatures and the public. For example, California's 1994 single-payor ballot initiative would have created a state constitutional right to a specified level of nurse staffing.[84]

Managed Care Organizations

Interprofessional relationships have also been dramatically changed by the rapid growth of managed care, which emphasizes prepayment and coordinated care. For example, closed-panel health maintenance organizations (HMOs) such as Kaiser-Permanente have long traditions of using nurse practitioners and physician assistants as primary care providers.[85] In addition to the now-ubiquitous utilization review nurse, managed care organizations also frequently employ or contract with nurses for health promotion activities, telephone consultations, and triage. Moreover, increases in physician employment (as opposed to self-employment), and even unionization, are adding to the common ground between physicians and other health professionals.[86]

The RAND Corporation recently conducted a study of nurse practitioners and physician assistants in group practices and HMOs.[87] In the settings evaluated, these providers worked collaboratively with physicians, demonstrated considerable flexibility in performance of specific tasks, and, in many instances, served as primary care practitioners for patients. Conflicts between health professionals over practice boundaries may be less frequent and less intense in institutional settings because the division of labor is determined collectively, preconceptions are replaced by experience, and working relationships that improve overall efficiency are rewarded. An Institute of Medicine study of two West Coast HMOs similarly revealed significant utilization of nurse practitioners and physician assistants.[88] In one mature HMO, adding a midlevel practitioner to a primary care physician's practice increased the physician's estimated catchment population from 1,800 to 2,700 persons.[89]

The cost advantage of nonphysician primary care practitioners appears to extend beyond direct compensation. Studies have shown that advanced practice nurses order fewer tests and perform fewer procedures than physicians, without any difference in outcome, apparently because of their practice philosophy and training.[90] It remains to be seen whether these differences will persist once physicians have learned to work under managed care incentives, and nonphysician practitioners have become accustomed to roles of greater authority.

The emergence of new organizations may further alter traditional relationships. For example, some group practices are experimenting with a combination of advanced practice nurse gatekeeping and specialty physician services. Managed mental health care has brought psychologists and, to some extent, social workers into networks with psychiatrists in order to meet the price demands of purchasers. Pharmaceutical firms are entering the clinical marketplace with "disease management" programs that rely on teams of advanced practice nurses, nutritionists, and other allied health professionals as well as physicians.

One cautionary note is that advanced practice nurses and physician assistants have been encouraged by government and tolerated by the medical profession in part because of a perceived shortage of physicians. However, selective contracting, primary care gatekeeping, and risk-sharing arrangements are now revealing *excess* capacity in many physician markets. Managed care plans have therefore been able to negotiate discounts on physician services, reducing the direct cost advantage of nonphysician practitioners.[91]

In addition, rapid growth and aggressive price competition have favored broad provider networks such as independent practice associations over more capital-intensive forms of managed care such as closed-panel HMOs.[92] Because these linkages often lack any institutional history of cooperative practice among different health professionals, they may exclude professionals other than physicians. For example, physician gatekeepers rarely refer patients to chiropractors.[93] Organized medicine has also lobbied to curtail practice privileges of professionals whom it perceives as rivals, although physician entrepreneurship and opposition from employers have somewhat diluted its influence.[94]

Healthcare Quality and Consumerism

Quality assurance and protection of the public have been the traditional justifications for licensure laws, scope of practice restrictions, and other legal limitations on the health professions.[95] However, the terms of the quality debate are changing. Not only are regulatory definitions recognized as imperfect surrogates for healthcare quality, but provider perceptions of quality are no longer accorded the degree of deference typical of a generation ago.[96]

The rise of large healthcare organizations has accelerated this process by increasing both information availability and public skepticism. Larson notes that medicine's professional sovereignty was due in part to the privacy of the doctor-patient transaction and the patient's consequent lack of quality-related information beyond his or her own uninformed conclusions and the opinions of other physicians.[97] Information on clinical practices is now routinely gathered, analyzed, and used by purchasers, private accrediting bodies (such as the National Committee on Quality Assurance), and government. Aided by the revolution in computing and telecommunications, many such entities are making data available to individual consumers. A survey of healthcare websites on the Internet is ample evidence of the public's appetite for and understanding of quality-related information.

Moreover, regard for patient autonomy—well recognized for leading bioethicists to question medical heroics—has also encouraged diversity of healthcare.[98] Patients are freer to explore practitioners who match their personal philosophies; for example, feminism and environmentalism have renewed interest in midwifery and naturopathy.[99] Legal limitations on access to these services have on occasion even prompted patient claims that state regulation of the health professions infringes constitutionally protected privacy rights.[100]

Given these trends, and a political climate favoring privatization of governmental functions, strict adherence to a traditional licensing approach may no longer be justified by concerns about quality. For example, voluntary certification may be a viable alternative to legal restrictions on practice for many health professionals. Certification and accreditation programs—such as medical specialty boards—are well established in healthcare, and could be adapted to provide consumers with accurate, timely information about health professionals.

A middle ground between restrictions on scope of practice and voluntary certification might limit the performance of certain hazardous activities to licensed health professionals. However, licensure would merely ensure "title protection"—the right to be called a "physician," "nurse practitioner," "pharmacist," or the like—while scope of practice would be unlimited. As is currently the case for physicians, the right to conduct specific activities could be in the credentialing discretion of each health professional's practice institution or managed care network, guided by private certification and accreditation organizations.

A more general issue presented by the rise of prepaid corporate healthcare is whether the traditional regulatory focus on individual practitioners should be supplanted entirely by some form of institutional licensure, allowing organizations to police their internal operations but holding them accountable for failures of oversight.[101] The paradigm of unmonitored, solo physician practice upon which licensure standards are based has virtually disappeared.[102] Most contemporary healthcare is collaborative, with multiple layers of support, peer review, and institutional oversight. Even in relatively isolated communities, advances in computing and communications are enabling primary care practitioners to obtain information and assistance from other health professionals via telemedicine.

High-quality managed care will require interdisciplinary skills and coordination, with providers of various professions assuming complementary roles in larger healthcare organizations. Efficiency considerations favor giving these organizations flexibility to accomplish their goals as cost-effectively as possible. As a practical matter, evidence suggests that legal restrictions on scope of practice are seldom determinative of actual behavior in large healthcare organizations. Instead, organizations tend to assign tasks flexibly—sometimes in disregard of the law—relying on internal quality controls to safeguard patients.[103]

Studies comparing advanced practice nurses and physician assistants to physicians have not shown differences in quality in situations within the claimed competence of each profession.[104] As Andrews observes, "the fact that the patients of physician assistants and advanced practice nurses fare as well as those of physicians indicates that these alternative providers accurately perceive the limits of their abilities and refer complicated patients to physicians."[105] Under these circumstances, direct government regulation of individual professionals may be less important to public safety than organizational resources, financial incentives, internal lines of authority, and institutional quality control.

An important determinant of success in any institutional oversight mechanism will be the stability of organizational structures. One problem with individual licensure has been the inability of resource-constrained public bodies to oversee large numbers of mobile professionals. A smaller universe of established organizations with greater interests in avoiding reputational injury and the financial resources to assist regulators in gathering and processing information might well be easier to monitor. However, the current trend toward "virtual integration" and the proliferation of transient, poorly capitalized enterprises would tend in the opposite direction.

A related issue is liability for patient injury. Legal accountability for patient injury has focused on physicians. For example, traditional tort doctrines held physicians responsible for negligent acts of supporting professionals, such as nurses, whether or not those professionals were employed by the physician.[106] However, malpractice liability in interdisciplinary practice may be unpredictable, exposing various classes of professionals to allegations of improper delegation or inadequate supervision as well as errors in diagnosis or treatment. Successful collaborative models therefore require a mechanism for liability to be shared, apportioned, or assumed by a third party such as a healthcare institution, without unduly sacrificing deterrence or jeopardizing compensation for injury. Moreover, the market for malpractice insurance will have to accommodate these changes.

Ethical Obligations and Public Service

Although much of this chapter has addressed economic influences on interprofessional relationships, most views of the health professions reject economic reductionism. For example, the "ideal of service"—a social contract to serve the public interest without regard to pay—is an important attribute of professionalism.[107] In today's world, that means both traditional good works and the demonstration of independence— at least in patient care and public health matters—from the business imperatives of managed care.

Many clinical and administrative approaches used by managed care organizations attempt to bridge the gap between individual patient benefit and population health management. Ascertaining the proper relationship between clinical judgment and patient advocacy is an important challenge for health professionals, particularly those taking on expanded responsibilities. Although several recent commentaries have explored the ethical effect of managed care on physicians and the physician-patient relationship, few have discussed its effect on other health professionals or the relationship among health professions.[108]

For example, the laying on of hands and the intimacy of the provider-patient relationship are closely linked to ethical precepts for healthcare professionals. In a managed care system, less expensive providers than physicians may be able to offer "high touch" care at reasonable cost.[109] If advanced practice nurses, physician assistants, and other health professionals are the people with whom patients have the most direct contact, patients may come to regard them as they do physicians today. This is potentially a weighty burden for health professionals accustomed to more insulated roles.

At the same time, many physicians (and nurses) now find themselves in supervisory and management roles less connected with hands-on patient care.[110] Upholding ethical obligations when discharging administrative duties in corporate environments may be difficult.[111] The public is also unaccustomed to viewing physicians in this light. In one case, a court dismissed out of hand the opinion of an insurance company's medical director, remarking that "[her] training is not only in medicine but in 'cost containment.' In which of these disciplines she is better trained would be an interesting question."[112] Suggestions have even been made to create an entirely new health profession, the patient advocate, to balance the systemwide responsibilities that physicians often assume in managed care.[113]

Finally, the social responsibilities of health professionals include caring for underserved populations. More than 40 million Americans, mainly low-income workers and their families, lack health insurance. According to a variety of studies, uninsured individuals receive less care and are in poorer health than insured individuals.

The cost-unlimited environment that prevailed until recently created "trickle-down" opportunities for other health professionals to fill service needs in geographic and specialty areas not considered desirable by physicians. Medicaid reimbursement policies and other special government programs assisted this process in order to expand access to care for underserved communities. As a result, nurse practitioners and physician assistants became the principal providers of primary care in many rural areas and inner cities, as did nurse-midwives and nurse anesthetists in their areas of competence.[114]

Factors in addition to economics may be responsible for this phenomenon.[115] For example, nursing education emphasizes public health and a holistic approach to patients, which may be more compatible with practice in general community clinics than in high-technology, specialized environments. Diversity of background may also contribute. Because preparation as a physician assistant or advanced practice nurse is shorter and less expensive than medical training, it has been more accessible to minorities and economically disadvantaged individuals, who are also more likely to practice in underserved areas. However, nonphysician providers are far from a panacea for the uninsured; many of the same economic and personal factors that discourage physicians also deter other health professionals, and lack of physician support is an additional drawback.

The regulation of interdisciplinary practice therefore has important implications for equity in the healthcare system. Narrow scopes of practice, restrictive reimbursement standards, and other legal barriers may limit access to care for large numbers of Americans. In the absence of a national commitment to universal health insurance, the potential for nonphysician practitioners to supply much-needed general health services at reasonable cost should not be ignored.

Conclusion

This chapter has described the regulation of interdisciplinary practice as it evolved during an era of physician hegemony and as it has begun to accommodate today's more cost-constrained medical marketplace. These developments can be interpreted in stark economic terms, but also reflect important ethical and public policy considerations, many of which go to the essence of professionalism in modern society.

Brint distinguishes between two models of professionalism: "social trustee professionalism," based on commitments to community stability and public service; and "expert knowledge professionalism," based on mastery of specialized information and technical skills.[116] The former is vulnerable to social change and devaluation, the latter to economic change and commodification. Both paradigms are evident in the history of interdisciplinary practice: legally sanctioned physician control justified by the rapid expansion of medical knowledge, organizational challenges to that control in response to economic imperatives, and the reemergence of social stewardship as a professional ideal.

The pace of change in the U.S. healthcare system and the pluralistic character of that system are additional obstacles to rational regulation of interdisciplinary practice. The role of law as a conservative force therefore raises an important question: to what degree should the legal system act as a restraint on a rapidly evolving marketplace? On one hand, concern for patient rights and public safety suggests caution in regulatory innovation. On the other, current laws constitute something of a Gordian knot, limiting opportunities for many health professionals, denying underserved populations access to qualified providers, and impeding the development of truly collaborative practice.

Considering the unpredictability of industry change, flexibility and vigilance are likely to be more valuable than regulatory detail or ideological consistency. Legal intervention may be needed, however, to deal with transitional issues created by the process of change, whatever its ultimate direction. Appropriate measures might include standardizing terminology, coordinating practices across jurisdictions, protecting vulnerable populations, and funding demonstration projects and evaluations research.

In the end, law has its limits—especially where ingrained professional cultures and practices are concerned. Whatever the law does or fails to do, meaningful improvements in interprofessional relations will probably have to wait until a new generation of health professionals has been trained in the changing ways of the world.

Acknowledgment

Supported in part by a grant from the Pew Charitable Trusts. The authors thank Janice Kam and Rosemary Auth for research assistance.

Notes

1. Physician Payment Review Commission (PPRC). 1995. *1995 Annual Report to Congress*. Washington, DC: PPRC.

2. Advanced practice nurses (nurses with master's degrees or the equivalent) and physician assistants (college graduates with at least one year of additional training) are sometimes referred to collectively as "midlevel practitioners," reflecting roles and responsibilities greater than those of registered nurses but less than those of physicians. There were approximately 139,000 advanced practice nurses in the United States in 1992: 58,000 clinical nurse specialists, 48,000 nurse practitioners, 7,400 certified nurse-midwives, and 25,000 nurse-anesthetists. Approximately 13,000 physician assistants were practicing nationally in 1995. M. S. Donaldson, K. D. Yordy, K. N. Lohr, and N. A. Vanselow (eds.). 1996. Institute of Medicine, *Primary Care: America's Health in a New Era*. Washington, DC: National Academy Press, 6-7–6-10. See also P. E. Jones and J. F. Cawley. 1994. "Physician Assistants and Health System Reform: Clinical Capabilities, Practice Activities, and Potential

Roles." *Journal of the American Medical Association* 271 (16): 1266. Most nurse practitioners work in outpatient settings as employees of hospitals, HMOs, or private physician practices. Similarly, the majority of physician assistants are employed in ambulatory settings, with about one-half providing primary care and one-quarter serving as surgical specialists. PPRC. 1994. *1994 Annual Report to Congress.* Washington, DC: PPRC, 267. Like physicians, most advanced practice nurses and physician assistants serve as points of entry for patients accessing the healthcare system.

3. "Limited license practitioners"—doctoral-level health professionals who provide clinical services of limited scope—also include dentists, oral surgeons, pharmacists, optometrists, and others. IOM, *Primary Care*, 5-16–5-18.

4. Nursing is the largest health profession, with 2.2 million licensed registered nurses as of March 1992. E. B. Moses. 1994. *The Registered Nurse Population: Findings from the National Sample Survey of Registered Nurses, March 1992.* Washington, DC: U.S. Government Printing Office. Nursing is also the most heterogeneous health profession, counting among its members junior-college graduates working as registered nurses as well as holders of master's or doctoral degrees serving as advanced practice nurses. Some traditional nursing functions are also performed by lesser-trained licensed vocational or licensed practical nurses, by nurses' aides, and by "unlicensed assistive personnel."

5. The preamble to the 1947 constitution of the World Health Organization (WHO) asserts that "Health is a state of complete physical, mental, and social well-being and not merely the absence of disease or infirmity." By redefining health in positive, moral terms, the WHO statement confirmed a trend toward medicalizing human suffering and identifying healthcare as the primary human good. D. Callahan. 1987. *Setting Limits: Medical Goals in an Aging Society.* New York: Simon & Shuster.

6. Several excellent books and articles describe the legal landscape affecting different classes of health professionals. See, e.g., B. R. Furrow, T. L. Greaney, S. H. Johnson, T. S. Jost, and R. L. Schwartz. 1995. *Health Law.* St. Paul, MN: West Publishing, 55–90; D. J. Mason, S. W. Talbot, and J. K. Leavitt (eds.). 1993. *Policy and Politics for Nurses: Action and Change in the Workplace, Government, Organizations and Community,* 2nd edit. Philadelphia, PA: W. B. Saunders; B. J. Safriet. 1992. "Health Care Dollars and Regulatory Sense: The Role of Advanced Practice Nursing." *Yale Journal on Regulation* 9 (2): 417–88; B. J. Safriet. 1994. "Impediments to Progress in Health Care Workforce Policy: License and Practice Laws." *Inquiry* 31 (1): 310–17; L. B. Andrews. 1996. "The Shadow Health Care System: Regulation of Alternative Health Care Providers." *Houston Law Review* 32 (5): 1273.

7. California alone regulates the following health professions in addition to medicine and nursing: chiropractors, clinical laboratory technicians, dentists, podiatric medicine, drugless practitioners, licensed midwives, research psychoanalysts, speech-language pathologists and audiologists, registered dispensing opticians, occupational therapists, dietitians, perfusionists, physical therapists, physical therapist assistants, nurse-midwives, nurse-anesthetists, nurse-practitioners, vocational nurses, psychologists, hearing aid dispensers, physician assistants, osteopathic physician assistants, osteopathic medicine, respiratory therapists, nursing home administrators, pharmacy, medical device retailers, psychiatric

technicians, veterinary medicine, acupuncturists, marriage, family and child counselors, and social workers. Andrews, "Shadow Health Care System."

8. G. J. Stigler. 1971. "The Theory of Economic Regulation." *Bell Journal of Economics and Management Science* 2 (1): 3; W. Gellhorn. 1976. "The Abuse of Occupational Licensing." *University of Chicago Law Review* 44 (1): 6.

9. E.g., Cal. Bus. & Prof. Code § 2051 (1996) (defining the practice of medicine); § 2052 (unauthorized practice).

10. See, e.g., E. Freidson. 1970. *Profession of Medicine*. New York: Dodd, Mead & Co.

11. National Council of State Boards of Nursing. 1995. *The Regulation of Advanced Practice Registered Nurses* Chicago: National Council of State Boards of Nursing, Inc.

12. E.g., N.Y. Educ. L. § 6951 (McKinney 1996); N.Y. Comp. Codes R. & Regs. tit. 10, § 20.1 et seq. (1996) (defining the practice of certified nurse-midwives).

13. E.g., N.Y. Educ. L. § 6542 (McKinney 1996); N.Y. Comp. Codes R. & Regs. tit. 10, § 94.2 (1996) (defining the practice of physician assistants).

14. Cal. Code Regs., tit. 16, § 302 (1996).

15. C. S. Weissert. 1996. "The Political Context of State Regulation of the Health Professions." In *The U.S. Health Workforce: Power, Politics, and Policy*, edited by M. Osterweis, C. J. McLaughlin, H. R. Manasse, Jr., and C. L. Hopper. Washington, DC: Association of Academic Health Centers, 81–91.

16. For example, California's attorney general recently interpreted the state's Nursing Practice Act as prohibiting nurse-midwives from performing episiotomies as "assisting of childbirth by . . . artificial, forcible or mechanical means," even though the act specifically provided for training of nurse-midwives to perform episiotomies and the Board of Registered Nursing had earlier stated that the procedure was part of the routine management of uncomplicated birth. 78 Op. Atty. Gen. Cal. 247, No. 94–1011 (July 31, 1995). See also H. W. Haggard. 1929. *Devils, Drugs, and Doctors*. New York: Harper & Bros. (describing the invention of the obstetrical forceps, which was kept secret by a family of physicians for over a century in order to control midwife training); R. W. Wertz and D. C. Wertz. 1989. *Lying-In: A History of Childbirth in America*. New Haven, CT: Yale University Press.

17. See *Virginia Academy of Clinical Psychologists v. Blue Shield of Virginia*, 624 F.2d 476 (4th Cir. 1980) (clinical psychologists); *Sandefur v. Cherry*, 547 F. Supp. 418 (M.D. La. 1982) (optometrists); *Pennsylvania Dental Hygienists' Association, Inc. v. State Board of Dentistry*, 672 A.2d 414 (Comm. Ct. Pa. 1996) (dental hygienists).

18. J. Kreplick. 1995. "Unlicensed Hospital Assistive Personnel: Efficiency or Liability?" *Journal of Health and Hospital Law* 28 (5): 292 (study suggesting that registered nurses spend as much as one-half their time on tasks suitable for unlicensed workers).

19. E.g., Cal. Bus. & Prof. Code §§ 2827, 2833.5 (Deering 1996) (certified nurse-anesthetists may provide anesthesia services to medical, dental, and podiatric patients, but may not "practice medicine or surgery").

20. *Oklahoma Board of Nursing v. St. John Medical Center* (unpublished decision granting injunctive relief to the Oklahoma board of nursing against a medical

center for using trained but unlicensed workers to place intravenous catheters and monitor cardiac rhythms).

21. E.g., *New York State Nurses Association v. Axelrod*, 544 N.Y.S. 2d 236 (N.Y. App. Div. 1989) (granting standing to professional association to challenge state regulations permitting licensed practical nurses to administer intravenous therapy); *Ohio Nurses Association, Inc. v. State Board of Nursing Education and Nurse Registration*, 540 N.E. 2d 1354 (Ohio 1989) (upholding procedural challenge to state's "position paper" granting licensed practical nurses the right to administer intravenous fluids).

22. Intergovernmental Health Policy Project. 1994. *Scope of Practice: An Overview of State Legislative Activity*. Washington, DC: George Washington University.

23. J. C. Kany. 1996. "Developing Rational Health Professions Licensure," in *The U.S. Health Workforce*, 107–19 (describing Maine Licensure Development Project).

24. E. H. Hadley. 1989. "Nurses and Prescriptive Authority: A Legal and Economic Analysis." *American Journal of Law & Medicine* 15 (2): 245.

25. M. Beck. 1995. "Improving America's Health Care: Authorizing Independent Prescriptive Privileges for Advanced Practice Nurses." *University of San Francisco Law Review* 29 (4): 951.

26. According to IMS America, midlevel practitioners accounted for 0.57 percent of prescriptions in April 1996, compared to 0.22 percent in 1992. "Nonphysician Prescribing Doubles." *American Medical News*, June 17, 1996, 2.

27. N.Y. Educ. L. § 6950 et seq. (McKinney 1996).

28. Courts have not dealt consistently with revisions to established professional classifications. In an analogous case in Connecticut, the court held that the establishment of strict requirements for physician-supervised nurse-midwives did not reflect legislative intent to outlaw independent practice by lay midwives. *Department of Public Health v. Vidam*, Pet. No. 930205-00-004 (Conn. Dept. Pub. Health, July 5, 1996).

29. IOM, *Primary Care*, 6-17–6-18.

30. Pew Health Professions Commission, L. J. Finocchio, C. M. Dower, T. McMahon, C. M. Gragnola, and the Taskforce on Health Care Workforce Regulation. 1995. *Reforming Health Care Workforce Regulation: Policy Considerations for the 21st Century*. San Francisco: Pew Health Professions Commission.

31. Ibid., 10.

32. L. S. Bohnen. 1994. *Regulated Health Professions Act: A Practical Guide*. Aurora, Ontario: Canada Law Book.

33. J. F. Cawley. 1996. "The Evolution of New Health Professions: A History of Physician Assistants," in *U.S. Health Workforce*, 189–207.

34. H. Taylor. 1996. "When Labor Meets Law: Midwives in Limbo." *Times Union* (Albany, NY), 10 March: 3.

35. American Nurses Association. 1993. *Registered Professional Nurses and Unlicensed Assistive Personnel*. Washington, DC: American Nurses Publishing.

36. E.g., Standards for Registered Nurse Teaching and Delegation to Unlicensed Personnel, Or. Admin. R. 851-45-011 (1988); 1994. "Connecticut Sets Practice Guidelines." 14 *NOCA Prof. Reg. News* 14 (November): 2.

37. National Council of State Boards of Nursing. 1995. *The Regulation of Advanced*

Practice Registered Nurses. Chicago: National Council of State Boards of Nusing, Inc.

38. *Best v. North Carolina State Board of Dental Examiners*, 423 S.E. 2d 330 (N.C. App. 1992), rev. denied 428 S.E.2d 184 (N.C. 1993) (state board of dental examiners, not board of nursing, has final authority to determine who is a "lawfully qualified nurse" to administer intraoral anesthetics).

39. Pew Commission, *Reforming Health Care Workforce Regulation*, 14–17.

40. Va. Code Ann. § 54.1-2507 (Michie 1996).

41. Pew Commission, *Reforming Health Care Workforce Regulation*, 29–34.

42. PPRC, *1994 Annual Report*, 274–75.

43. E.g., Washington State Department of Health, Mandatory Malpractice Insurance Coverage for Health Care Practitioners, January 1995.

44. S. D. Cohn. 1989. "Professional Liability Insurance and Nurse-Midwifery Practice." In *Medical Professional Liability and the Delivery of Obstetrical Care*, vol. 2, edited by V. P. Rostow and R. J. Bulger. Washington, DC: National Academy Press.

45. G. A. Robinson. 1986. "Midwifery and Malpractice Insurance: A Profession Fights for Survival." *University of Pennsylvania Law Review* 134: 1001.

46. *Wilk v. American Medical Association*, 895 F.2d 352 (7th Cir. 1990), cert. denied, 496 U.S. 927 (1990).

47. E.g., *Virginia Academy of Clinical Psychologists v. Blue Shield*, 624 F. 2d 476 (4th Cir. 1980), cert. denied, 450 U.S. 916 (1981) (finding plan policy to exclude psychologists unlawful restraint of trade).

48. E.g., *Bhan v. NME Hospitals, Inc.*, 929 F. 2d 1404 (9th Cir. 1991), cert. denied, 502 U.S. 994 (1991) (granting summary judgment to hospital that had decided to grant staff privileges to physician anesthesiologists but not to nurse-anesthetists).

49. M. A. Hall and G. F. Anderson. 1992. "Health Insurers' Assessment of Medical Necessity." *University of Pennsylvania Law Review* 140 (5): 1637.

50. E.g., *Tudor v. Metropolitan Life Insurance Co.*, 539 N.Y.S.2d 690 (N.Y. Dist. Ct., Nassau Cty. 1989) ("It should not be necessary in order to justify reimbursement for medical expenses that a patient be required to satisfy a committee, a board, or produce a plethora of testimonials from the mainstream of the medical establishment.").

51. E.g., Fla. Stat. 627.6403 (1996) (acupuncturists); Minn. Stat. 43A.316 (1995) (applying to public employers); Va. Code Ann. 38.2-4221 (1996) (mandating payment to several classes of professionals if coverage includes services within their licenses).

52. E.g., Cal. Ins. Code §§ 10127.3, 11512.12 (requiring insurers and HMOs to offer coverage of acupuncture); N.Y. S.B. 5972 (1995) (bill vetoed by Governor requiring coverage of chiropractic services).

53. 29 U.S.C. § 1101 et seq. (1996).

54. See, e.g., *Hayden v. Blue Cross and Blue Shield of Alabama*, 855 F. Supp. 344 (M.D. Ala. 1994) (Alabama law requiring direct payment of nurse-anesthetists preempted by ERISA).

55. Compare *CIGNA Healthplan v. Louisiana* ex rel. Ieyoub, 82 F.3d 642, (5th Cir. 1996) (holding any-willing-provider law preempted by ERISA) with *Stuart Circle*

Hospital Corp. v. Aetna Health Management, 995 F.2d 500 (4th Cir.), cert. denied, 510 U.S. 1003 (1993) (determining that Virginia any-willing-provider statute was a law regulating insurance and therefore saved from preemption).

56. Cf. Joint Commission on Accreditation of Healthcare Organizations. 1995. *Certification and Accreditation Manual For Hospitals*. Chicago: JCAHO, HR. 1., 358 (requiring processes to ensure adequate staffing, compliance with law, and continual oversight and assessment).

57. Cf. *Cook v. Workers' Compensation Department*, 758 P. 2d 854 (Or. 1988).

58. 42 U.S.C. § 1395x(r) (1996).

59. See, e.g., 42 U.S.C. §§ 1395k(a), 1395x(s) (1996).

60. PPRC, *1994 Annual Report*, 283–84.

61. 42 U.S.C. §§ 1396d(a)(17), (21) (1996).

62. 42 U.S.C. §§ 1396d(e), (g) (1996).

63. E.g., Ark. Stat. Ann. 17-87-311 (1995) (advanced practice nurses and nurse practitioners); Cal. Welfare & Institutions Code § 14132 (1996) (chiropractors, podiatrists, psychologists, and others); Fla. Stat. 409.908 (1995) (nurse practitioners, chiropractors, and podiatrists).

64. E.g., *Yapalater v. Bates*, 494 F. Supp. 1349 (S.D.N.Y. 1980); aff'd, 644 F.2d 131 (2d Cir. 1981), cert. denied, 455 U.S. 908 (1982) (state not required to reimburse psychiatrist for services of employed psychologists, social workers, nurses, and behavioral therapists where such personnel were not practicing medicine as defined by state law).

65. See, e.g., 42 U.S.C. § 1395b-1 (1996) (providing grants to study cost-effectiveness of nurse practitioners and physician assistants).

66. IOM, *Primary Care*, 7-14–7-17.

67. L. H. Aiken and M. E. Gwyther. 1995. "Medicare Funding of Nurse Education: The Case for Policy Change." *Journal of the American Medical Association* 273 (19): 1528.

68. *Dent v. West Virginia*, 129 U.S. 114 (1889) (West Virginia statute that requires every practitioner of medicine to be certified in that state does not deprive practitioner of estate or interest in the profession without due process of law). Cf. U.S. General Accounting Office. *Health Care Access: Innovative Programs Using Nonphysicians*, GAO/HRD-93-128 (Washington, DC: GAO, 1993) (describing federal health programs that employ healthcare professionals subject to federal laws and directives).

69. Health Security Act, H.R. 3600, 103d Cong., 1st Sess., § 1161 (1993).

70. Pew Commission, *Reforming Health Care Workforce Regulation*, 1–8.

71. PPRC, *1994 Annual Report*, 281–83.

72. Mont. Uniform Professional Licensing and Regulatory Procedures, § 37-1: 301–19 (1995).

73. See PPRC, *1995 Annual Report*, 135–52. However, economic protectionism is inducing some states to heighten rather than ease restrictions on licensure given the potential for telemedicine. E.g., Tex. H.B. 2669 (1995) (declaring that treatment by electronic media of patients located in Texas is practice of medicine in Texas).

74. R. Briffault and S. Glied. "Federalism and the Future of Health Care Reform" in

The Privatization of Health Care Reform, edited by G. Bloche. Oxford University Press (forthcoming).

75. A. Abbott. 1989. *The System of Professions: An Essay on the Division of Expert Labor*. Chicago: University of Chicago Press.

76. As Larson has observed, for many decades the organization of American medicine maximized the effectiveness of producer associations such as physician self-regulatory groups because "the sum of individual consumers are not, and most probably cannot, [*sic*] be organized." M. S. Larson. 1977. *The Rise of Professionalism: A Sociological Analysis*. Berkeley, CA: University of California Press, 23. This changed in the 1980s when employers self-funded ERISA plans, overcame decades of docile acceptance of healthcare cost increases, and evolved into organized purchasers of healthcare. PPRC, *1995 Annual Report*, at 187–89.

77. K. D. Yordy. 1996. "The Nursing Workforce in a Time of Change," in *The U.S. Health Care Workforce*, 141–52.

78. L. H. Aiken, J. Sochalski, and G. F. Anderson. 1996. "Downsizing the Hospital Nursing Workforce." *Health Affairs* 15 (4): 88–92.

79. The average income of a nurse practitioner was approximately $44,000 in 1992 compared with $110,000 for a family practice physician. A nurse-midwife earned about $44,000 annually and a nurse-anesthetist $76,000, while an obstetrician earned $200,000 and an anesthesiologist $220,000. E. B. Moses, *Registered Nurse Population*; PPRC, *1995 Annual Report*, 305–7.

80. J. Cromwell. 1996. "Health Professions Substitution: A Case Study of Anesthesia." in *U.S. Healthcare Workforce*, 219–28.

81. R. Riportella-Muller, D. Libby, and D. Kindig. 1995. "The Substitution of Physician Assistants and Nurse Practitioners for Physician Residents in Teaching Hospitals." *Health Affairs* 14 (2): 181; B. A. Green and T. Johnson. 1995. "Replacing Residents with Midlevel Practitioners: A New York City–Area Analysis." *Health Affairs* 14 (2): 192.

82. B. R. Alper and S. O. Miller. 1995. "Unions, Nurses, and the Health Care Industry: Recent Administrative and Judicial Developments." *Journal of Health and Hospital Law* 28 (2): 65.

83. Recent National Labor Relations Board (NLRB) decisions have rejected challenges to the inclusion of charge nurses in collective bargaining units, distinguishing the exercise of independent judgment in one's individual professional capacity from the exercise of judgment as a supervisor of other employees on behalf of an employer. E.g., Providence Hosp., Case No. 19-RC-12866, 320 N.L.R.B. 49 (Jan. 3, 1996), Nyamed, Inc., Case No. 3-RC-10166, 320 N.L.R.B. 65 (Feb. 2, 1966) (holding that charge nurses are not "supervisors" under the National Labor Relations Act). However, these situations are likely to become more difficult to resolve as the line blurs between managerial and clinical roles, and more professionals perform administrative functions. See also *NLRB v. Health Care & Retirement Corporation*, 511 U.S. 571 (1994) (overturning the NLRB's previous test, under which nurse supervisory activity incidental to treatment of patients was not considered exercised in the interest of the employer).

84. Cal. Prop. 186 (1994). A similar provision was contained in a failed 1996 initiative (Prop. 216), along with strict limitations on firing healthcare workers and a tax on

hospitals that merge. M. Schwartz. 1996. "Battle over California HMOs Heads for Showdown at Polls." *The Press-Enterprise* (Riverside, CA), 6 August: D3.

85. K. Bell and J. Mill. 1989. "Certified Nurse-Midwife Effectiveness in the Health Maintenance Organization Obstetric Team." *Obstetrics and Gynecology* 74 (1): 112.

86. In 1994, 42.3 percent of physicians were employees of hospitals, HMOs, or other corporate entities. P. R. Kletke, D. W. Emmons, and K. D. Gillis. "Current Trends in Physicians' Practice Arrangements: From Owners to Employees." 1996. *Journal of the American Medical Association* 276 (7): 555. See also 1996. "Doctors Looking to Unions as Managed Care Makes Gains." *American Medical News* (Sept. 23/30). A counterweight is that most states prohibit as a formal matter the corporate practice of medicine, including the employment of physicians under some circumstances, and at least six states still actively enforce those prohibitions. Corporate practice laws have even been revitalized in some states in reaction to the increase in competitive pressures in healthcare. See, e.g., *Berlin v. Sarah Bush Lincoln Health Center*, 664 N.E.2d 337 (Ill. App. Ct. 1996) (voiding employment contract between physician and nonprofit hospital in suit challenging hospital's enforcement of noncompetition provision).

87. PPRC, *1994 Annual Report*, 269–72.

88. R. M. Scheffler. 1996. "Life in the Kaleidoscope: The Impact of Managed Care on the U.S. Health Care Workforce and a New Model for the Delivery of Primary Care," in IOM, *Primary Care*, at Appendix E.

89. D. A. Kindig. 1996. Federal Regulation and Market Forces in Physician Workforce Management, in *The U.S. Health Care Workforce*, 47–56.

90. S. McGrath. 1990. "The Cost-Effectiveness of Nurse Practitioners." *Nurse Practitioner* 15 (7): 40–42.

91. Cf. *United Food and Commercial Workers, Local 555 v. Kaiser Foundation Hosps., Inc.*, 1996 WL 89365, No. 95-1145-FR (D. Or. Feb. 23, 1996) (unionized radiology technicians alleged that an HMO plan to have physicians and physician-supervised nurses perform ultrasound examinations was a violation of the technicians' collective bargaining agreement).

92. R. A. Berenson. 1997. "Beyond Competition." *Health Affairs* 16 (2): 171–80.

93. R. Berg. 1993. "HMO Exclusion of Chiropractors." *Southern California Law Review* 66 (2): 807.

94. Scheffler, "Kaleidoscope."

95. Cf. C. H. Baron. 1983. "Licensure of Health Care Professionals: The Consumer's Case for Abolition." *American Journal of Law & Medicine* 9 (3): 335 (the resulting restrictions of consumer choice have long been apparent).

96. Larson, *Rise of Professionalism*, 24, 32–33 (physicians differentiated themselves from other consulting professions through a successful "negotiation of cognitive exclusiveness"; i.e., by establishing scientific communities inaccessible to the general public).

97. Ibid.

98. Managed care has reversed some of these trends by limiting patients' choices of providers. Medical savings accounts, which would entitle individual consumers to spend pretax dollars on a wide variety of health interventions as long as they

purchase a high-deductible insurance policy as well, might be a counterweight. See K. E. Thorpe. 1995. "Medical Savings Accounts: Design and Policy Issues." *Health Affairs* 14 (3): 254.

99. So-called "alternative medical providers" are frequently overlooked in discussions of the health professions. Some of these individuals are licensed, such as acupuncturists, while many are not. Public investment in alternative medicine is substantial and increasing. One in three Americans used unconventional therapies in 1991, spending a total of $13.7 billion. G. Kolata. 1996. "On Fringes of Health Care, Untested Therapies Thrive." *New York Times,* 17 June: A1, col. 1.

100. B. A. McCormick. 1983. "Childbearing and Nurse-Midwives: A Woman's Right to Choose." *New York University Law Review* 58 (3): 661. See, e.g., *State v. Kimpel,* 665 So.2d 990 (Ala. Crim. App. 1995), cert. denied, 116 S. Ct. 674, 133 L. Ed.2d 523 (1995) (letting stand state court ruling that state's interest in regulating midwifery outweighed privacy right of potential patient).

101. See Pew Commission, *Reforming Health Care Workforce Regulation,* 12. See also Hadley, "Prescriptive Authority," 297; Andrews, "Shadow System," 1304; R. J. Carlson. 1970. "Health Manpower Licensing and Emerging Institutional Responsibility for the Quality of Care." *Law and Contemporary Problems* 35 (4): 849.

102. Only 29.3 percent of physicians were in solo practice in 1994, compared to 40.5 percent as recently as 1983. Kletke et al., "Current Trends."

103. PPRC, *1994 Annual Report,* 103.

104. E.g., L. Baldwin, T. Raine, L. Jenkins, G. Hart, and R. Rosenblatt. 1994. "Do Providers Adhere to ACOG Standards? The Case of Prenatal Care." *Obstetrics and Gynecology* 84 (4): 549 (finding that nurse-midwives more frequently adhere to the standard of care than obstetricians or family physicians). See also S. A. Brown and D. E. Grimes. 1993. *Nurse Practitioners and Certified Nurse-Midwives: A Meta-Analysis of Studies of Nurses in Primary Care Roles.* Washington, DC: American Nurses Publishing; Office of Technology Assessment, U.S. Congress. 1986. *Health Technology Case Study 37, Nurse Practitioners, Physician Assistants, and Certified Nurse-Midwives: A Policy Analysis.*

105. Andrews, "Shadow System," 1285.

106. Nurses' professional skills and obligations were ignored in early malpractice cases, which tended to absolve them of professional negligence if they had followed a physician's order, unless the danger of that order would have been apparent to a layperson. *Byrd v. Marion General Hospital,* 162 S.E. 738 (N.C. 1932); E. J. Armstrong. 1987. "Nurse Malpractice in North Carolina: The Standard of Care." *North Carolina Law Review* 65 (3): 579. Other professionals who worked in subservient roles to physicians, such as physician assistants, were treated similarly.

107. See, e.g., R. Pound. 1953. *The Lawyer from Antiquity to Modern Times.* St. Paul, MN: West Publishing Co. (defining a profession as "pursuing a learned art as a common calling in the spirit of public service . . .").

108. D. Blumenthal. 1996. "Effect of Market Reforms on Doctors and Their Patients." *Health Affairs* 15 (2): 172; R. A. Scott, L. H. Aiken, D. Mechanic, and J. Moravcsik. 1995. "Organizational Aspects of Caring." *Milbank Quarterly* 73 (1): 77.

109. Andrews, "Shadow System."

110. Nurses have traditionally labored under multiple and occasionally conflicting

duties to patients, supervising physicians, and institutional employers. Armstrong, "Nurse Malpractice."

111. For a discussion of the ethical dilemmas of managers, see R. Jackall. 1988. *Moral Mazes: The World of Corporate Managers*. New York: Oxford University Press.

112. *Florence Nightingale Nursing Service, Inc. v. Blue Cross & Blue Shield of Alabama*, 832 F. Supp. 1456, 1461 (N.D. Ala. 1993), aff'd, 41 F.3d 1476 (11th Cir. 1995), cert. denied, 115 S. Ct. 2002, 131 L. Ed.2d 1003 (1995).

113. See M. Mehlman. 1996. "Medical Advocates: A Call for a New Profession." *Widener Topics in Law 1996* 1 (1): 299.

114. Nearly 19 percent of certified nurse-midwives provide care in high-poverty areas, compared to 10 percent of obstetrician-gynecologists. PPRC, *1994 Annual Report*, 273–78; Institute of Medicine. 1989. *Prenatal Care: Reaching Mothers, Reaching Infants*. Washington, DC: National Academy Press.

115. Andrews, "Shadow System."

116. S. Brint. 1994. *In an Age of Experts: The Changing Role of Professionals in Politics and Public Life*. Princeton, NJ: Princeton University Press.

5

ADMINISTRATIVE LAW ISSUES IN
PROFESSIONAL REGULATION

Eleanor Kinney

THIS CHAPTER examines the major administrative law issues facing state boards that regulate the health professions, the professionals those boards regulate, and the public they protect.[1] Specifically, this chapter addresses the procedures that guide the work of these boards, for the business of administrative law is the procedures by which government agencies execute the responsibilities that the legislature assigns in enabling legislation. The nature of an agency's statutory assignments, in general, dictates the content of the procedures that guide its work.

State licensure boards are charged with implementing the professional practice acts that define the scope of practice for the particular regulated health profession, other professional responsibilities, and proscribed conduct subject to discipline.[2] Traditionally, state licensure boards for all health professions have had three specific statutory assignments. The first is to control entry into the profession through examination and licensure. The second is to monitor and discipline licensees who violate the profession's practice act or standards of professional conduct. The third and overarching responsibility is to protect the public from healthcare professionals whose services are unsafe or of poor quality.

Since the 1970s, which saw marked increases in the frequency and severity of medical malpractice lawsuits,[3] policymakers, consumer representatives, and the health professions have increasingly criticized the performance of state licensure boards in protecting the public from incompetent practitioners and poor quality healthcare.[4] Out of a similar concern for maintaining the quality of care in federal health insurance programs, the inspector general of the U.S. Department of Health and Human Services has likewise exhibited considerable interest in the operation and procedures of state licensure boards.[5] As a result of these developments, state licensure boards have become much more proactive in their role of protecting consumers against deficient practitioners.[6] Specifically, state licensure boards have focused greater efforts on ferreting out incompetent practitioners.[7] Nevertheless, the bulk of state board disciplinary actions continue to concern criminal violations and substance abuse impairment.[8]

Another, more recent challenge to state licensure boards comes from another quarter. A revolution has occurred in the way the healthcare industry approaches the assessment and improvement of quality healthcare. Specifically, quality assessment has moved from emphasis on the process by which care is delivered and enforcement of process standards to the emphasis on holding healthcare providers accountable for the outcomes of care.[9] Much of this move has been influenced by TQM theory, which stresses work standardization to reduce errors and measures quality in terms of customer satisfaction and other client-oriented outcome measures.[10]

The fallout of this quality revolution for state licensure boards is pressure on boards to expand their functions to include improving the quality of practitioner services through the public dissemination of data and information about healthcare professionals.[11] Assumption of this quality improvement function is possible because of advances in computer technology that enable state boards to collect and maintain detailed information about practitioners.[12] These data can be used to advise consumers about poor quality practitioners and also to identify practitioners whose conduct warrants further discipline particularly for incompetence.

However, this quality improvement function is quite different from traditional licensure and discipline functions. A central question is whether this new function of quality improvement through data collection and dissemination is truly compatible with the culture of state boards that have evolved by implementing markedly different functions such as prosecution of quasi-criminal offenses. To the extent that the functions of state licensure boards are so expanded, the mission and culture of state boards must be reevaluated. Indeed, the internal structure and operation of state boards are implicated, as are the procedures by which state boards organize and execute their responsibilities.

The Nature of Procedure

Procedure has been defined as the "mode of proceeding by which a legal right is enforced, as distinguished from the substantive law which gives or defines the right. . . ."[13] Procedure pertains to the form, manner, or order of conducting legal and regulatory business. While it does not have anything to do with the content or purpose of a regulatory scheme, it has everything to do with how expeditiously and fairly that regulation is executed and enforced, particularly with respect to private individuals.

Historically, when government enforces law or regulation against private parties, the elements of requisite procedure depend on the seriousness of the consequences of successful enforcement for regulated parties. In criminal proceedings, in which the stakes for the prosecuted are quite high, the federal Constitution and most state constitutions require fairly rigorous procedural protections. When the consequences of an agency action are nonspecific, such as in promulgating a general rule that applies to all regulated parties, the procedural protections for affected individuals are quite minimal.[14] Further, administrative procedures must also facilitate execution of legislatively assigned responsibilities with minimal staff and resources. But one guiding principle is clear: the content and scope of procedures depend directly on the purpose, consequences, and intrusiveness of the agency function. This principle has critical implications for state licensure boards because of the nature of their traditional functions—licensure and discipline—and because of the newer and different function of quality improvement.

The traditional function of licensure involves the development and administration of examinations and the adjudication of applications for licenses. The basic theory of licensure is limiting market entry to those practitioners with demonstrated competence in order to protect the public from unsafe and poor quality professional services. The licensure process is relatively straightforward and generally involves an adjudication of whether to grant a license to an individual applicant. Nevertheless, the consequences of licensure are crucial to individual applicants. Thus, the associated procedures must assure regular and fair determinations.

The second traditional function of discipline is of a criminal nature. The theory of the discipline function is to identify and eliminate the "bad apples" from the profession. The prohibitions giving rise to discipline generally pertain to professional misuse of drugs, impairment due to drug or alcohol abuse, sexual misconduct with patients, and conviction of crimes. The procedures of state licensure boards in investigating and prosecuting these infractions are really quasi-criminal as they pertain to the adjudication of infractions of specific prohibitions. State discipline statutes also authorize discipline on competency grounds. The concept of competence contemplates a pattern of many problems—which may be relatively inconsequential in isolation—but which are problematic collectively. Discipline for breaches of professional competence, while not really criminal in nature, has such serious implications for the charged professional that disciplinary proceedings for incompetence generally command the use of procedures comparable to those used for criminal infractions.

The quality improvement function is fundamentally different than disciplining infractions of specific prohibitions. Quality improvement involves the collection and publication of data on past professional performance as well as outcomes of care for individual practitioners. The theory of quality improvement is that disclosure of information enables consumers to make informed choices and avoid poor quality providers. The availability of usable data—made possible by advances in computer technology—poses particularly difficult challenges to state boards that assume multiple, diverse, and arguably inconsistent functions.

Organizational Structure of State Licensure Boards

Under prevailing administrative law theory, the legislature creates an administrative agency or assigns responsibilities to existing agencies to execute the laws it has enacted. To execute the law effectively, agencies must have authority to make rules and policies to delineate specifically the content of statutory standards and requirements. Agencies must also have authority to adjudicate disputes between agencies and resistant regulated parties that arise when agencies seek to enforce the statutory and regulatory requirements. Further, agencies must have authority to obtain information from regulated parties in order to execute the agencies' statutory responsibilities and protect the public.

In most states, licensure boards are composed chiefly of members of the regulated profession who are appointed by the governor. In response to criticism that professionally dominated boards with little oversight are not aggressive in discharging their disciplinary functions against professional colleagues,[15] states have changed board composition requirements and increased the number of "public" nonpractitioner members.[16] Also, some states have changed the location of state licensure boards in the organization of state government to make state licensure boards more efficient and effective and also to exert control over professionally dominated boards.[17] Specifically, those states have moved boards into departments of state government that often include licensure and disciplinary boards for other professions. Nevertheless, despite this movement for organizational reform, the autonomous licensure board remains the dominant organizational model.

As a matter of federal constitutional law, states have considerable latitude in the composition of state licensure boards. In *Friedman v. Rogers*,[18] the United States Supreme Court upheld a Texas statute specifying that the state's optometry board be composed of a majority of optometrists from a particular school of optometrists that fundamentally opposed the way in which the plaintiff optometrist practiced. The Court essentially concluded that the plaintiff optometrist had no constitutional right to be regulated by optometrists of a persuasion similar to one's own.

The organizational structure of state licensure boards is an especially important issue, given the disparate functions that state boards are now assuming and the constraints on staff and resources that face state agencies.[19] Specifically, the boards should be organized in such a way that the same staff do not perform different, inconsistent functions such as the collection and dissemination of data on practitioners with a view toward improving quality of care on the one hand and developing the case against practitioners prosecuted in disciplinary proceedings on the other. Regardless of the so-called combination of functions problem described below, the organizational structure of state boards must accommodate the performance of different assignments generally through different divisions of the agency and certainly with different staff.

Rule Making and Policymaking

Rule making is the exercise of delegated legislative power.[20] Through rule making, agencies interpret their enabling statutes and also establish specific requirements of regulatory programs mandated by statute. Under administrative law orthodoxy, rules can only have legislative effect if they are promulgated according to statutory rule-making procedures.[21] Rule making plays an important role in delineating and publicizing how an agency will exercise the discretion accorded in a broadly drafted enabling statute. Most state licensure and discipline statutes contain express authorization for rule making.[22]

State licensure boards promulgate rules to address almost every aspect of their work. Specifically, rules set forth standards, criteria for enforcing standards, definitions of unprofessional conduct, license eligibility requirements, requirements for competency assessments, procedures for disciplinary proceedings, and procedures for information management, and they address a host of other matters.[23] Indeed, the importance of rule making for the work of state licensure boards cannot be overestimated.[24] As one observer stated,

> Rulemaking [*sic*] underlies the entire operation of the licensing board. . . . Though statutes describe general expectations for implementation, it is up to the board to make the expectations operational through specific requirements and procedures.[25]

Most states have state administrative procedure acts that establish rule-making procedures for legislative rules, and govern if the board's enabling statute is silent on rule-making procedures. The federal constitution does not require oral hearings or other detailed procedures on federal or state agency rule making as a matter of procedural due process.[26] Most state administrative procedure statutes, which are based on the Commission on Uniform State Laws' Model State Administrative Procedure Act (MSAPA) for either 1961 and 1981, set forth rule-making procedures.[27] State administrative procedure act (APA) rule-making procedures, however, are not always as streamlined as informal rule-making procedures under the federal APA, which simply requires agencies to give notice of the content of a proposed rule and an opportunity to comment.[28] For example, many states impose additional procedural requirements, such as oral hearings or appeals to administrative law judges, on their informal rule-making procedures.[29] Even the MSAPA requires agencies to give advanced notice of the rule making and state the text of the proposed rule in full.[30]

Rule making has not been a particularly controversial issue with respect to state licensure boards. Courts have generally upheld the authority of state licensure boards to promulgate rules on a variety of issues.[31] For example, in *Levy v. Board of Regulation and Discipline in Medicine,*[32] involving the revocation of a license upon a criminal conviction for healthcare fraud, the court upheld the authority of the licensure board to promulgate a regulation making conviction of a crime a basis for disciplinary action despite the silence of the enabling statute on the subject.

As state boards take on additional functions, including the collection and dissemination of data on healthcare professionals for quality improvement and consumer protection, rule making can play an important role. Specifically, through rule making, boards can delineate the types of data to require from professionals and can also specify procedures for the reporting, collecting, maintaining, and disseminating of data. The development and specification of policy on these data and other important issues through rule making may assuage concerns within the regulated profession and the public about the board's expanded functions, or at least about how the board will exercise its discretion in executing new as well as traditional functions.

Adjudication

Adjudication is the exercise of delegated judicial power.[33] Adjudication involves agency decisions to apply a statute, regulation, or policy to individual private parties. State licensure boards make several types of adjudications, which reflect their multiple substantive functions. First, they make decisions to grant licenses to practitioners upon demonstration of good character and successful examination results. Second, state licensure boards engage in disciplinary proceedings against practitioners who violate the applicable practice act or engage in conduct proscribed under the state's professional licensure and discipline laws. If the professionals disagree with the state board's decisions on these matters, they are generally entitled to an opportunity to challenge the board's action in an adjudicative proceeding.

State Statutory Requirements

State licensure and discipline statues generally require specific procedures characteristic of evidentiary hearings.[34] However, if the enabling statute is silent regarding such procedural requirements, the state administrative procedure act generally contains provisions regarding the conduct of adjudicative proceedings that would apply. The MSAPA, for example, establishes minimal procedures for adjudications involving licenses that comport with procedural due process requirements. Specifically, the MSAPA requires notice of the hearing, hearing procedures, and criteria for review of the boards decision by the courts.[35]

The model statute of the Federation of State Medical Boards contains detailed recommendations for adjudication procedures for disciplinary proceedings based on the general principle that "The medical practice act should provide for procedures that will permit the Board to take appropriate enforcement and disciplinary action as required, while assuring fairness and due process to licensees."[36] The Federation statute includes provision for notice of charges to the accused, an opportunity for a fair and impartial hearing for the accused before the board or its examining committee, an opportunity for representation by counsel as well as the presentation of testimony evidence and argument, subpoena power, and attendance of witnesses, and a record of the proceedings.[37]

The Federation model statute also includes specific authorization for judicial review of decisions in disciplinary proceedings.[38]

Many state licensure and disciplinary statutes expressly provide for emergency proceedings when a threat to public health is at stake.[39] Some state discipline statutes have special provisions such as summary suspension when the licensee has been convicted of, or pleads guilty to, narcotics violations and other serious crimes of moral turpitude.[40] Further, the MSAPA expressly authorizes summary suspension of licenses to protect public health and for comparable emergencies.[41] The Federation of State Medical Boards expressly recommends that state statutes contain authority for summary suspension and other emergency measures.[42]

Constitutional Requirements

The procedural due process clause of the federal constitution, applied to the states through the Fourteenth Amendment, requires administrative agencies to provide private parties notice and an opportunity to be heard if they have a protected property or liberty interest at stake and wish to challenge an adverse agency action affecting that protected interest.[43] Historically, the United States Supreme Court has regarded a license as a protected interest under the due process clause.[44] Further, most states have comparable due process clauses in their state constitutions, although few cases raise state constitutional due process guarantees. The United States Supreme Court has articulated what procedures are required as a matter of federal constitutional law. The basic requirements are fairly flexible but include at least adequate and timely notice of the charges, an opportunity to confront witnesses and present evidence, and an unbiased decision maker.[45] In *Mathews v. Eldridge*,[46] the Supreme Court established a three-prong test to determine if specific procedures meet due process requirements. Basically, the test involves a balancing of the private and public interest and the capability of the procedures in question to achieve an accurate decision.[47]

There is an extensive due process jurisprudence involving due process challenges to disciplinary proceedings of state licensure boards.[48] Indeed, several of the major decisions of the Supreme Court on the requirements of procedural due process for the adjudication of administrative disputes have involved state licensure boards. In addition to the basic requirements of notice and an opportunity to be heard, important and sometimes controversial due process issues include the nature of the decision maker, bias, the combination-of-functions problem, rights to discovery, evidentiary standards, and sanctions.

Notice and an Opportunity to Be Heard

Courts have invalidated board decisions on grounds that licensees did not have adequate notice of charges leveled against them.[49] However, courts have sustained state boards if boards have cured deficiencies in notice before the hearing.[50] Courts have generally required that hearings over the denial or termination of a professional license be evidentiary hearings on the record and with rights of cross-examination, to present evidence, and representation by counsel, as well as others features of evidentiary hearings.[51] Such evidentiary hearings are generally not required if the discipline is based on a prior criminal conviction,[52] a disciplinary decision of another state,[53] or on findings of another state agency.[54] In general, hearings must occur before sanctions and adverse actions are imposed. However, in cases involving threats to public health amounting to an emergency, agencies can act first and provide a subsequent opportunity to be heard.[55]

Nature of the Decision Maker

A crucial issue with respect to state licensure boards is the nature of the decision maker in adjudicative proceedings. Most state licensure boards use administrative law judges (ALJs) to conduct the disciplinary hearings, with the board itself ultimately deciding the case based on the ALJ's findings and conclusions.[56] In *Guerrero v. New Jersey*,[57] the United States Court of Appeals for the Third Circuit ruled that using ALJs to hear professional disciplinary matters ultimately decided by the board did not deny a practitioner due process or equal protection under the federal constitution.

Bias

Another important issue is bias on the part of the decision maker or board. This issue is particularly important for professionally dominated licensure boards that give the appearance of having decision makers that come to the proceeding with a particular point of view. Indeed, the United States Supreme Court's major decision on the bias issue involved a state licensure board. In *Gibson v. Berryhill*,[58] the United States Supreme Court found that a state licensure board was biased essentially because of its composition. Specifically, the state optometry board, which was composed exclusively of so-called professional optometrists who stead-fastly opposed the practice of optometry by commercial corporations, brought disciplinary actions against individual optometrists employed by a commercial optical company. The Court agreed with the plaintiff commercial optometrists that the board, which was dominated by professional optometrists, was biased by prejudgment and pecuniary interest and thus could not constitutionally be fair and impartial in hearings regarding revocation of optometrists' licenses.

Combination of Functions

The combination-of-functions problem results from the fact that the state licensure board has the responsibility of both prosecuting and adjudicating a disciplinary proceeding.[59] Again, the major decision of the United States Supreme Court on the combination-of-functions problem involved a state licensure board. In *Withrow v. Larkin*,[60] the Supreme Court rejected a due process claim and ruled that members of the state licensure board were not precluded from holding an adversary hearing on the matter of a possible license suspension on the basis of charges developed in the board's own investigation. Nevertheless, some courts remain uncomfortable with the Supreme Court's resolution of the combination-of-functions problem in *Withrow*.[61] It is noteworthy that the Federation of State Medical Boards' model statute contains an express recommendation on the separation of the investigative and judicial functions of state licensure boards in disciplinary proceedings.[62]

Right to Discovery

State cases have also addressed the rights of prosecuted professionals to discover evidence in the board's investigative file and have differed on the degree to which prosecuted licensees have access to investigative information.[63] Nearly all states require boards to disclose exculpatory information to charged practitioners.[64]

Evidentiary Standards

Evidentiary standards have been especially controversial in disciplinary proceedings before state licensure boards.[65] Basically at issue is the appropriate standard of evidence in disciplinary actions against practitioners: the "clear and convincing" standard used in quasi-criminal proceedings or the more lenient "preponderance of the evidence" standard used in most civil litigation. The preponderance-of-the-evidence standard requires proof supporting a finding that the existence of a contested fact is more probable than not, while the clear-and-convincing standard requires proof that the truth of the contested fact is highly probable.[66] The latter standard provides greater protection for practitioners, but adds complexity to the investigative process, and appears to make it less likely that a board will persevere on a case through a full evidentiary hearing.[67]

Often prosecuted practitioners have argued that a higher evidentiary standard is required as a matter of procedural due process. Several courts have rejected this analysis.[68] For example, in *In re Polk*,[69] the Supreme Court of New Jersey concluded that, given the government's interest to protect public health and the fact that only a showing of "flagrant" misconduct leads to discipline, a preponderance-of-the-evidence standard did not imperil procedural due process principles.[70]

As state licensure boards have become more proactive in identifying and disciplining errant professionals, many state legislatures have been persuaded to raise the evidentiary standard in professional disciplinary determinations.[71] On the other hand, to make it easier for state licensure boards to discipline practitioners, several states have adopted the preponderance-of-the-evidence standard and moved from the more rigorous clear-and-convincing standard.[72] The Federation of State Medical Boards recommends the preponderance-of-the-evidence standard in its model medical discipline statute.[73] Some states have gone even further to ease the evidentiary burden of the state licensure board in disciplinary proceedings. For example, Wisconsin has allowed a court finding of practitioner negligence in a medical malpractice case to serve as conclusive evidence before the licensure board.[74]

Use of Expert Testimony

Professional licensure boards have considerable authority in making their decisions regarding professional misconduct. Specifically, several courts have held that boards can make decisions based on their own professional judgment without the supporting, independent expert testimony.[75]

Sanctions and Remedies

In the exercise of their delegated judicial power, state licensure boards have the authority to impose sanctions on practitioners and provide other remedies as appropriate.[76] State practice acts generally accord state licensure boards a considerable range of sanctions against disciplined professionals.[77] These include final sanctions such as revocation of a license and a host of intermediate sanctions that can involve, for example, ongoing monitoring of a practice and required therapy in the case of an impaired practitioner.[78]

State boards are reluctant to impose the most onerous and final sanction of license revocation.[79] While the ultimate sanctions of the suspension or revocation of a license may be appropriate in the case of serious infractions of disciplinary prohibitions, these sanctions may be too strong in some cases. Consequently, state boards have developed and imposed a variety of intermediate sanctions such as required monitoring or continuing professional education.[80] Finally, a crucial issue, discussed below, is the confidentiality of sanctions and the degree to which the public should be informed that the board has imposed sanctions on a practitioner.[81]

Judicial Review

In administrative law theory, judicial review is the check against arbitrary or incorrect action by an administrative agency, and its availability justifies the delegation and combination of extensive powers within administrative agencies.[82] Disciplined practitioners view judicial review as a powerful source of protection against the perceived injustice of a state licensure board's action. Yet both state and federal courts have accorded the decisions of state licensure boards considerable deference in their adjudicative determinations and in the sanctions the boards impose.[83]

The Supreme Court has never established a right to judicial review as a matter of procedural due process.[84] In practice, however, every state has provided some form of judicial review function for decisions of state boards in disciplinary proceedings.[85] There is a large body of law that sets forth the criteria for the "availability" of judicial review of an agency action.[86] Judicial review is always available when the enabling statute expressly permits review. State licensure boards almost always provide for judicial review of their decisions in disciplinary actions against practitioners.[87] Further, the MSAPA would generally provide for judicial review if the enabling statute were silent on the availability of review.[88] It is noteworthy that the Federation of State Medical Boards expressly recommends availability of judicial review as a matter of fair process in disciplinary proceedings.[89]

The basic role of the court reviewing administrative agency decisions is to determine whether the agency complied with various legal standards in its decision making. The most important standards for judicial review—which have been adopted in MSAPA,[90] many state and federal statutes, and the federal APA[91]—are whether the agency's decision complied with the law; was not arbitrary, capricious, or an abuse of discretion; and, in a matter on the record such as an evidentiary hearing, was supported by substantial evidence.[92] Reviewing courts have generally accorded considerable deference to the decisions of state licensure boards in disciplinary matters,[93] although courts have often concluded that board decisions are not supported by substantial evidence.[94]

In general, judicial review of state licensure board decisions and rules has not been controversial.[95] One issue that has been controversial, however, is the propriety of judicial stays of the orders and sanctions of state boards pending judicial review.[96] State courts often issue such stays pending appeal to protect the professional's reputation and livelihood pending a possible exoneration.[97] However, judicial review often takes a long time and, in the meantime, a dangerous practitioner may continue to practice. Some state legislatures have taken measures to curb the latitude of state courts in granting stays of state licensure board disciplinary orders.[98] These limits range from outright bans on stays to the imposition of strict standards for the application of stays. Some states have given statutory priority to state licensure board decisions on the dockets of reviewing courts.[99]

Collection and Dissemination of Information

To execute their quality improvement and consumer protection responsibilities efficiently, licensure boards increasingly collect and disseminate data about the professionals whom they regulate. As one scholar aptly noted, "[i]nformation is the fuel on which the administrative engine operates."[100] With respect to their four major statutory assignments of licensure, enforcement, consumer protection, and quality improvement, state licensure boards obtain and use information in different and often conflicting ways. Consequently, the role of collector, creator, custodian, and potential source of information on practitioners poses enormous and controversial procedural challenges to state licensure boards.

Obtaining Information

In general, administrative agencies can obtain information regarding regulated parties in three ways: (1) required reports; (2) administrative inspections; and (3) subpoenas, which are generally imposed in the course of investigations and disciplinary proceedings. They can also collect information on regulated parties and the relevant industry through studies and other sources. State boards have extensive powers to investigate, including the express authority to issue subpoenas, in their enabling legislation.[101] Also, state boards require the reporting of extensive professional and personal information in the application for licensure and compel information about performance on qualifying examinations.

In the enforcement function, agencies must identify practitioners in need of discipline and then develop the cases against them in disciplinary proceedings before sanctions are imposed. State licensure boards get information primarily through consumer complaints, which is at best unsystematic and inefficient and at worst an unreliable way to ensure that a state board is concentrating its scarce investigative resources on the practitioners most in need of monitoring and discipline.[102] State boards are particularly limited in the way in which they obtain information to establish incompetence. They do not have systematic means for the surveillance of a professional practice to detect multiple errors in order to develop a sufficient record of incompetence.[103] State boards generally do not have the requisite cooperative working relationships with hospitals and professional liability insurers that would facilitate the reporting of problematic practitioners.[104] Further, practitioners are often reluctant to criticize other professionals for errors. However, many state professional discipline statutes authorize audits of practitioners' practices following the filing of a complaint in a disciplinary action.[105]

To address inadequacies in the way in which state licensure boards obtain information about problems with practitioners that warrant investigation and disciplinary action, states have increasingly imposed various reporting requirements on individuals and institutions, including hospitals and insurance companies as well as other practitioners, that have information about practitioner conduct.[106] Specifically, many states require professional liability insurers to report malpractice claims and outcomes and court clerks to report judgments in cases involving crimes, negligence, errors, or omissions in practice.[107] Some states require practitioners themselves to report to state licensure boards information on another practitioner's professional misconduct, alcoholism, drug addiction, or mental disability.[108] In sum, state licensure boards rely heavily on reporting requirements, as well as consumer complaints, to identify practitioners in need of discipline.

However, the procedures by which state boards compel information and the protections accorded regulated parties in disciplinary and other proceedings are highly dependent on the functions that the agency seeks to accomplish with the information. For example, a regulated party that is subject to an investigation in a quasi-criminal disciplinary proceeding ought to have more protections than a regulated party from whom information is requested in the course of a fairly benign proceeding such as rule making or publication of information for the benefit of the public—other crucial functions of administrative agencies. The concern arises when information is required and obtained in more benign proceedings, such as the reporting of information to a data bank used to prepare public reports, and is then used to establish the basis for investigation and possible prosecution in a disciplinary proceeding. For example, a case for incompetence might well be developed from information reported to the licensure board for other purposes. Health professionals are appropriately concerned about reporting requirements and the use of reported information.

The collection and dissemination of information about individual practitioners is crucial in the consumer protection function of state licensure boards. Consumers are protected when they are advised about board actions on licensure and discipline adjudications, as well as outcomes data and other data on practitioners generated from the new quality improvement function. Yet, with increased responsibilities to monitor and improve the quality of care of individual practitioners and to protect the public from poor quality practitioners, the information management function of state licensure boards has become much more complex. Now state boards are in a position to use the same information about individual practitioners for quality improvement and consumer protection purposes as well as for licensure and discipline.

When an agency, which also has quasi-criminal enforcement authorities, has the power to collect, maintain, and disseminate information—even for completely different and quite benign purposes—opportunities for the misuse of data arise. An important question is the extent to which these data can also be used in the investigation and prosecution of disciplinary proceedings. For example, would the doctrine of official notice, which allows administrative agencies to use information they have obtained regarding regulated parties in adjudicative proceedings,[109] enable state licensure boards to use data collected regarding practitioners as proof of issues in disciplinary proceedings?

Disseminating Information

State licensure boards disseminate information extensively in discharging their consumer protection responsibilities. Disseminating information about individual practitioners has become more prevalent as boards respond to pressure to minimize the professional dominance of the professional discipline process and provide more protection to consumers from unsafe practitioners. Now state licensure boards disseminate information about their licensure and disciplinary adjudications and, increasingly, data about the quality of a practitioner's professional care. To the extent that boards maintain accurate, complete, and current information, they can serve practitioners well as a source of accurate information for consumers, providers, and also managed care organizations that seek information on practitioners with whom they contract.

In general, states have increased public access to information and proceedings of all types due to the enactment of statutes in many states since the 1960s to open up government generally. State freedom of information acts have become almost universal,[110] although, in a few states, they do not apply to professional disciplinary hearings.[111] Many states have open records statutes that make public records available to consumers.[112] Also, many states have "open meeting" laws that require administrative proceedings to be conducted in public.[113] It is noteworthy that, in its model statute, the Federation of State Medical Boards recommends that license revocation and suspension proceedings be handled in an "open hearing" and that final decisions in disciplinary proceedings be a matter of public record.[114]

There has been considerable controversy regarding board disclosures about disciplinary proceedings. Historically, state boards have made it difficult for consumers to get information about practitioners and their disciplinary actions.[115] For example, many boards will not provide information about a disciplinary action over the telephone and require the inquirer to come to the board's office or submit a written request for information.[116] More recently, however, some states have taken innovative steps to inform the public about their deliberations regarding individual practitioners. For example, Massachusetts has created a practitioner database including disciplinary information that is accessible through the Internet, and plans to publish a practitioner profile directory.[117] Also, several states make information on disciplinary actions against health practitioners available to newspapers and other media outlets, including public libraries.[118] These approaches are consistent with the quality improvement functions that many state boards are adopting.

State licensure boards also report their actions to other national databases that serve as repositories of information about practitioners. The Federation of State Medical Boards maintains a voluntary database on the decisions of state licensure boards in disciplinary proceedings and is a major source of information for state boards about disciplinary actions against professionals in other states. However, many state boards do not report disciplinary actions consistently or enter into confidentiality agreements with disciplined practitioners that preclude the reporting of disciplinary actions.[119] Also, since the late 1980s, state licensure boards have also had to report their decisions to the National Practitioner Data Bank.[120]

The major users of data in these national databases are state licensure boards, hospital providers in the credentialing process, licensure boards in other states, and, increasingly, managed care companies in selecting practitioners with whom to contract. Consumer watchdog organizations use these national data banks to obtain and publicize information about disciplined practitioners. For example, the Public Health Research Group publishes a nationwide "questionable doctors report" that provides a state-by-state list of over 8,000 doctors disciplined by state and federal government agencies.[121]

A crucial issue from the consumer perspective is the degree of confidentiality to accord disciplinary proceedings. While there is consensus that the final orders and sanctions of disciplinary proceedings should be made public, there is debate about whether complaints, hearings, and other aspects of the disciplinary proceeding should be public. Practitioners understandably press for confidential proceedings because of the damage to their reputation and practice likely to be caused by the fact that a disciplinary action has been initiated against them. Further, some state professional licensure and discipline statutes provide for closed proceedings in some instances, primarily to protect the reputation of the licensee.[122]

Often state boards will enter into confidentiality agreements or agreements not to publicize disciplinary actions with practitioners in order to expedite the disciplinary action and impose the appropriate sanction on the practitioner.[123] Interestingly, while generally favoring open hearings and public decisions, the Federation of State Medical Boards' model statute does recommend an exemption to state open meeting laws to permit confidential conferences with accused licensees who seek or agree to such a conference.[124]

The decisions on the confidentiality of disciplinary proceedings before final adjudication are split, however. For example, in *Johnson Newspaper Corp. v. Melino*,[125] the Court of Appeals of New York ruled that the press did not have a right of access to a disciplinary proceeding, stating that "there is no suggestion that professional disciplinary hearings have any tradition of being open to the public and no show that public access plays 'a significant positive role' in the functioning of these proceedings."[126] In *Daily Gazette Co., Inc. v. West Virginia Board of Medicine*,[127] the media challenged the constitutionality of the confidentiality provisions of the state's medical practice act. The court agreed, ruling that the public had the right of access to the complaint, and the board's decision regarding the complaint, even if the board found that no probable cause existed for bringing the disciplinary action. The court concluded further that records of a hospital peer review committee that become part of the record in a board disciplinary action can also be disclosed if the board concludes that it has probable cause to proceed with the complaint.[128] In a subsequent decision, *Thompson v. West Virginia Board of Osteopathy*,[129] the Supreme Court of Appeals of West Virginia ruled a state board must issue findings of fact and conclusions of law that are available to the public along with the complaint, even if the board determines that there is no probable cause to proceed with the complaint.

At the heart of the debate over publication and disclosure is a thorny balance of interests. On the one hand is the public's need to know about potentially dangerous practitioners. On the other hand is the understandable concern of practitioners about privacy and the protection of their reputations. Clearly the balance should tip in favor of consumers with respect to final agency actions against providers. The balance should probably tip in favor of practitioners in the case of complaints that have yet to be adjudicated.

Conclusion

In general, the trend in the administrative law pertaining to the activities of state licensure boards is to make it easier for boards to execute their statutory responsibilities. This trend reflects criticism that state boards have not been vigorous enough in protecting the public from poorly qualified or outright dangerous practitioners. Nevertheless, concerns remain within the health professions about the need for greater procedural protections in the face of increasingly proactive and effective boards. The press for more demanding evidentiary standards in disciplinary proceedings, for example, is symptomatic of this general concern among health professionals.

The crucial issue of administrative law facing state licensure boards is the degree to which their important quasi-criminal functions inhibit the usefulness or even the appropriateness of their adopting other quality improvement functions that require state licensure boards to be custodians and disseminators of extensive information about practitioners' qualifications and performance to consumers and purchasers of healthcare services. On the one hand, state licensure boards could provide an important service in the management of information that managed care organizations use to select practitioners in a public and accountable manner. Such a role would be extremely helpful since managed care companies are now making private credentialing decisions about practitioners that have enormous implications for practitioners' access to patients and facilities. Indeed, in terms of regulation for the purposes of consumer protection, information dissemination may actually be more effective than aggressive enforcement against individual errant practitioners.

On the other hand, it may well be that the best and most important function of state licensure boards is the identification and elimination of "bad apples" from the profession. Although few practitioners are, fortunately, targeted in the disciplinary function, this function is absolutely crucial for the overall safety of the American public. Why is it not enough if state licensure boards do a good job adjudicating licensure and disciplining licensees for quasi-criminal conduct and incompetent professional practice?

To the degree that other functions are added to this critical responsibility, care must be given to the procedural implications of such an assignment. Professionals must be treated fairly in the licensure and discipline processes, and state licensure boards must be able to proceed as expeditiously and efficiently as possible in accomplishing their disciplinary responsibilities. The management of data on practitioners is the most tricky problem from a procedural perspective because state boards, in disciplinary proceedings, have great opportunities for improperly using data and information obtained in the quality assurance function. For example, if reported information from practitioners that is collected to be used chiefly to inform consumers about the relative quality of a practitioner's professional performance is used to establish grounds for initiating disciplinary proceedings, greater procedural protections are required in the collection and management of the information. Such procedures may impede the expeditious dissemination of information of interest to consumers.

Indeed, it may be inappropriate for boards to engage in quality improvement activities that involve extensive data collection and dissemination. These functions may not only be inconsistent with the traditional board functions from a procedural perspective but may be so fundamentally inconsistent that the same agency, given inevitable constraints in staff and resources, may not be able to make the requisite conceptual and cultural adaptation necessary to execute all these functions effectively. In sum, careful attention is needed in assigning and designing the functions of state licensure boards.

Notes

1. See B. R. Furrow, T. L. Greaney, S. H. Johnson, T. S. Jost, and R. L. Schwartz. 1995. *Health Law.* St. Paul, MN: West Publishing Company, 1; § 3-4-3-11, 90–108; T. S. Jost. 1995. "Oversight of the Quality of Medical Care: Regulation, Management, or the Market?" *Arizona Law Review* 37 (3): 825; J. Gross. 1984. *Of Foxes and Hen Houses: Licensing and the Health Professions.* Westport, CT: Quorum Books; F. P. Grad and N. Marti. 1979. *Physicians' Licensure and Discipline.* Dobbs Ferry, NY: Oceana Publications, Inc.; R. C. Derbyshire. *Medical Licensure and Discipline in the United States.* Westport, CT: Greenwood Press. See generally, M. Moran and

B. Wood. 1993. *States, Regulation and the Medical Profession*. Philadelphia, PA: Open University Press; R. D. Blair and S. Rubin. 1980. *Regulating the Professions*. Lexington, MA: D.C. Heath and Co.

2. For boards regulating physicians, the Federation of State Medical Boards of the United States has published a model practice statute for the medical profession and periodically publishes state-by-state tables on state adoption of selected provisions of state medical practice acts. Federation of State Medical Boards of the United States, Inc. 1994. *A Guide to the Essentials of a Modern Medical Practice Act*, 7th edit. Fort Worth, TX: Federation of State Medical Boards of the United States, Inc.; The Federation of State Medical Boards of the United States, Inc. 1995. *Exchange, 1995–1996*. Fort Worth, TX: The Federation of State Medical Boards of the United States, Inc.

3. V. R. Posner. 1986. "Trends in Medical Malpractice Insurance, 1970–1985." *Law and Contemporary Problems* 49 (2): 57.

4. See, e.g., Council on Medical Education. 1988. "Report on Medical Licensure." *Journal of the American Medical Association* 259 (13): 1994; AARP, Health Advocacy Services Program Department. 1987. *Effective Physician Oversight: Prescription for Medical Licensing Board Reform*. Washington, DC: AARP; S. Wolfe et al. 1985. *Medical Malpractice: The Need for Disciplinary, Not Tort Reform*. Washington, DC: Public Citizens Research Group.

5. Office of the Inspector General, U.S. Department of Health and Human Services. 1993. *State Medical Boards and Quality of Care Cases: Promising Approaches*. Washington, DC: DHHS; Office of the Inspector General, U.S. Department of Health and Human Services. 1991. *Performance Indicators, Annual Reports, and State Medical Discipline: A State-by-State Review*. Washington, DC: DHHS; Office of the Inspector General, U.S. Department of Health and Human Services. 1989. *State Medical Boards and Medical Discipline*. Washington, DC: DHHS.

6. Jost, "Oversight of the Quality of Medical Care," 831–35.

7. OIG, *State Medical Boards*, 18; Gross, 16.

8. OIG, *State Medical Boards*, 15; T. S. Jost. "Oversight of the Quality of Medical Care," 862. See also T. S. Jost, Linda Mulcahy, Stephen Strasser, and Larry A. Sachs. 1993. "Consumers, Complaints, and Professional Discipline: A Look at Medical Licensure Boards." *Health Matrix* 3 (Summer): 309 (an empirical study of the work of medical licensure boards).

9. See, e.g., D. M. Berwick. 1989. "Continuous Quality Improvement as an Ideal in Health Care." *New England Journal of Medicine* 320 (1): 53; D. M. Berwick, A. B. Godfrey, and J. Roessner. 1990. *Curing Health Care: New Strategies for Quality Improvement*. San Francisco: Jossey-Bass; G. Laffel and D. Blumenthal. 1989. "The Case for Using Industrial Quality Management Science in Health Care Organizations." *Journal of the American Medical Association* 262 (20): 2869.

10. See, e.g., W. E. Deming. 1986. *Out of Crisis*. Cambridge, MA: Massachusetts Institute of Technology; W. E. Deming. 1993. *The New Economics for Industry, Government, Education*. Cambridge, MA: Massachusetts Institute of Technology; J. M. Juran. 1989. *Juran on Leadership for Quality: An Executive Handbook*. New York: The Free Press.

11. Jost, "Oversight of the Quality of Medical Care," 851–53; OIG, *State Medical Boards*, 18–20. See Gross, *Of Foxes and Hen Houses*, 135–59.

12. Jost, "Oversight of the Quality of Medical Care," 864.

13. Black's Law Dictionary, "Procedure," 1203 (6th ed. 1990).

14. See B. Schwartz. 1996. *Administrative Law*. Boston: Little, Brown and Company; § 1-7, at 15.

15. See OIG, *State Medical Boards*, 10; Gross, *Of Foxes and Hen Houses*, 94.

16. OIG, *State Medical Boards*, 10; Grad and Marti, *Physicians' Licensure*, 58; Gross, *Of Foxes and Hen Houses*, 97.

17. Gross, *Of Foxes and Hen Houses*, 97.

18. 440 U.S. 1 (1978).

19. See R. Cohen and M. Rose. 1993. *Allocation of Decision Making Authority Between Board Members and Staff: Ten Case Studies by the Citizen Advocacy Center*. Washington, DC: Citizen Advocacy Center.

20. K. Davis and R. Pierce. 1994. *Administrative Law*, vol. 1 3rd edit. Boston: Little Brown and Company; § 7.1, at 287.

21. Ibid. § 7.1, at 288.

22. W. Morris. 1984. *Revocation of Professional Licenses by Government Agencies*. Charlottesville, VA: The Michie Company; § 2-2, at 19.

23. Gross, *Of Foxes and Hen Houses*, 102, Morris, *Revocation*, § 2-2, at 18-23.

24. Because of the importance of rule making to state licensure boards, the National Association of Attorneys General has written a manual on rule-making procedures for state licensure boards. See National Association of Attorneys General. 1978. *Rulemaking Manual for Occupational Licensing Boards*. Washington, DC: National Association of Attorneys General. See Gross, *Of Foxes and Hen Houses*, 102.

25. Ibid., 101–2.

26. See, e.g., *United States v. Florida East Coast Ry.*, 410 U.S. 224 (1973); *Bi-Metallic Co. Colorado*, 239 U.S. 441 (1915).

27. Model State Administrative Procedure Act, 1981 Act (U.L.A), § 3-103, Model State Administrative Procedure Act, 1961 Act (U.L.A), § 2. See A. E. Bonfield. 1986. *State Administrative Rulemaking*. Boston, MA: Little Brown and Company; § 1.2, at 4-11.

28. 5 U.S.C. § 553 (1994).

29. Bonfield, *State Administrative Rulemaking*, §§ 6.4–6.6, at 180–232.

30. Model State Administrative Procedure Act, 1981 Act (U.L.A.) § 3-103; Model State Administrative Procedure Act, 1961 Act (U.L.A.) § 5.

31. See, e.g., *Department of Professional Regulation v. Durrani*, 455 So.2d 515 (Fla. App. 1984); *Levy v. Board of Registration and Discipline*, 392 N.E.2d 1936 (Mass. 1979). See Morris, *Revocation*, § 2-2, at 19.

32. 392 N.E.2d 1036, 1038-39 (Mass. 1979).

33. Schwartz, *Administrative Law*, § 2.18, at 74.

34. Furrow et al., *Health Law* § 3-13, at 109; Morris, *Revocation*, §§ 5-4–5-10, at 100–23; Grad and Marti, *Physicians' Licensure*, 144.

35. Model State Administrative Procedure Act, 1981 Act (U.L.A.) § 4-101–4-102; Model State Administrative Procedure Act, 1961 Act (U.L.A.) § 1(4), 9, 10, 15 et seq.

36. Federation of State Medical Boards of the United States, Inc. *Guide*, Section X.

37. Ibid.

38. Ibid.

39. Furrow et al., *Health Law*, § 6-5(c), at 387–90; Morris, *Revocation*, § 5.8 at 113; Grad and Marti, *Physicians' Licensure*, 120.

40. Morris, *Revocation*, § 3.3, at 36; Grad and Marti, *Physicians' Licensure*, 130.

41. Model State Administrative Procedure Act, 1981 Act (U.L.A.) § 4-501; Model State Administrative Procedure Act, 1961 Act (U.L.A.) § 14(c).

42. Federation of State Medical Boards of the United States, Inc. *Guide*, Section X.

43. See, e.g., *Dent v. State of West Virginia*, 129 U.S. 114, (1889); *Fleury v. Clayton*, 847 F.2d 1229 (7th Cir. 1988); *Mishler v. Nevada State Board of Medical Examiners*, 896 F.2d 408 (9th Cir. 1990); *Dayoub v. Commonwealth*, 453 A.2d 751 (Pa. 1982). See Schwartz, *Administrative Law*, §§ 5.1-5.2, at 225; Morris, *Revocation*, § 5-6, at 106; Furrow et al., *Health Law*, § 3-13, at 109.

44. *Ex parte Robinson*, 19 Wall. 505, 512 (U.S. 1874); *Schware v. Board of Bar Examiners*, 353 U.S. 232 (1957); *Gilchrist v. Bierring*, 14 N.W.2d 724 (Iowa 1944); *State v. State Medical Board*, 20 N.W. 238 (Minn. 1884). See Schwartz, *Administrative Law*, § 5.12, at 249.

45. *Goldberg v. Kelly*, 397 U.S. 254 (1970); *Goss v. Lopez*, 419 U.S. 565 (1976).

46. 424 U.S. 319 (1976).

47. 424 U.S., at 321.

48. Morris, *Revocation*, §§ 5-1–5-10, at 65-121; Grad and Marti, *Physicians' Licensure*, 141–77. These two older works include an excellent and detailed review of the law of procedural due process as it pertains to state licensure boards. For a more recent treatment of the subject, see Furrow et al. *Health Law* §§ 3-13–3-18, at 109–13.

49. See Furrow et al. *Health Law* 1, § 3-14, at 109, citing *Celaya v. Department of Professional Regulation*, 560 So.2d 382 (Fla. App. 1990); *Wagman v. Florida Board of Medicine*, 590 So.2d 12 (Fla. App. 1991); *Willner v. Department of Professional Regulation, Board of Medicine* 563 So.2d 805 (Fla. App. 1990); *In re Magee*, 362 S.E.2d 564 (N.C. App. 1987). See also Morris, *Revocation*, §§ 5-1–5-5, at 65-109; Grad and Marti, *Physicians' Licensure*, 149.

50. See Furrow et al., *Health Law*, 1, § 3-14, at 110, citing *In re Jones*, 590 N.E.2d 72 (Ohio App. 1990); *Arkansas State Medical Board v. Leipzig*, 770 S.W.2d 661 (Ark. 1989).

51. *Mahmoodian v. United Hospital Center, Inc.*, 404 S.E.2d 750 (W. Va. 1991). See also Furrow et al., *Health Law*, § 3-17, at 73; Morris, *Revocation*, §§ 5-5–5-6, at 102–4; Grad and Marti, *Physicians' Licensure*, 144.

52. Furrow et al., *Health Law*, 1, § 3-15, at 110, citing *Galang v. State*, 484 N.W.2d 375 (Wis. App. 1992); *Paiano v. Sobol*, 572 N.Y.S.2d 440 (App. 1991) *Dragan v. Commissioner*, 530 N.Y.S.2d 896 (App. 1988). See also Morris, *Revocation*, §§ 5-6, at 105; Grad and Marti, *Physicians' Licensure*, 144.

53. Furrow et al., *Health Law*, 1, § 3-17, at 111, citing *In the Matter of Cole*, 476 A.2d 836 (N.J. Super. App. Div. 1984); *McKay v. Bd.*, 788 P.2d 476 (Or. App. 1990). See also Grad and Marti, *Physicians' Licensure*, 146.

54. Furrow et al., *Health Law*, 1, § 3-17, at 111, citing *Camperlengo v. Barell*, 578 N.Y.S.2d 504, 585 N.E.2d 504 (App. 1991); *Choi v. State*, 550 N.Y.S.2d 267, 549 N.E.2d 469 (App. 1989); *Abraham v. Ambach*, 522 N.Y.S.2d, 318 (App. 1987).

55. Schwartz, *Administrative Law*, § 5-10, at 244; Furrow et al., *Health Law*, 1, § 1-17, at 34.

56. See Grad and Marti, *Physicians' Licensure*, 154.

57. 643 F.2d 148, 149 (3d Cir. 1981).

58. 411 U.S. 564 (1973).

59. Furrow et al., *Health Law*, 1, § 3-18, at 111–12, citing *Lyness v. Commonwealth*, 605 A.2d 1204 (Pa. 1992); *Bruteyn v. State Dental Council and Examining Board*, 380 A.2d 497 (Pa. 1977). See also Morris, *Revocation*, § 5.3, at 87; Grad and Marti, *Physicians' Licensure*, 148.

60. 421 U.S. 35 (1975). See also *Cooper v. State Board of Medicine*, 623 A.2d 433 (Pa. 1993); *Tighe v. Commonwealth*, 397 A.2d 1261 (Pa. 1979). See Furrow et al., § 3-18, at 111–13; Morris, *Revocation*, § 5-3, 87–99.

61. See, e.g., *Lyness v. Commonwealth*, 605 A.2d 1204 (Pa. 1992); *Rogers v. Texas Optometry Board*, 609 S.W.2d 248 (Texas 1980); *Goldberg v. Commonwealth*, 410 A.2d 413 (Pa. 1979); *Bruteyn v. Commonwealth*, 380 A.2d 497 (Pa. 1977). See Furrow et al., *Health Law*, 1, § 3-17, at 112–13.

62. Federation of State Medical Boards of the United States, Inc. *Guide*, Section X.

63. Furrow et al., *Health Law*, 1, § 3-16, at 110, citing *Wills v. Composite Board*, 384 S.E.2d 636 (Ga. 1989); *Board v. Spinden*, 798 S.W.2d 472 (Mo. App. 1990); *Rojas v. Sobol*, 563 N.Y.S.2d 284 (App. 1990); *Smith v. Department of Registration*, 120 Ill.Dec. 360, 523 N.E.2d 1271 (Ill. App. 1988). See also Morris, *Revocation*, § 5-1, at 66; Grad and Marti, *Physicians' Licensure*, 141.

64. Furrow et al., *Health Law*, § 3-16, at 110.

65. OIG, *State Medical Boards*, 9–10.

66. C. McCormick and J. Strong. (eds.). 1992. *McCormick on Evidence*, 4th edit. St. Paul, MN: West Publishing Co. § 339, at 575.

67. OIG, *State Medical Boards*, 9.

68. See, e.g., *In re Polk*, 449 A.2d 7 (N.J. 1982); *Eaves v. Board of Medical Examiners*, 467 N.W.2d 234 (Iowa 1991); *Rucker v. Michigan Board of Medicine*, 360 N.W.2d 154 (Mich. App. 1984). Citizen Advocacy Center. 1992. *A Resource Guide for Responding to Attempts to Weaken State Medical Licensing Boards by Legislating a Higher Standard of Evidence*. Washington, DC: AARP, 8–9.

69. 449 A.2d 7 (N.J. 1982).

70. 447 A.2d, at 12–14.

71. Citizen Advocacy Center, *Legislating a Higher Standard of Evidence*.

72. See Federation of State Medical Boards of the United States Inc., *Exchange*; § 3, at 72 (Table 23); Citizen Advocacy Center, *Legislating a Higher Standard of Evidence*, 8–10.

73. Federation of State Medical Boards of the United States, Inc. *Guide*, Section X, 14.

74. Ibid.

75. See, e.g., *In re Griffith*, 585 N.E.2d 937 (Ohio App. 1991); *Arlen v. State Medical*

Board, 399 N.E.2d 1251 (1980). But see *Sizemore v. Board of Dental Examiners*, 747 S.W.2d 389 (Tex. App. 1987).

76. See Schwartz, *Administrative Law*, §§ 2-25–2-26, at 90–94; Grad and Marti, *Physicians' Licensure*, 173–76.

77. For example, the federation recommends that state licensure boards have the following sanctions available in disciplining physicians: revocation, suspension, or both; probation; censure; reprimand; fines; and payments of disciplinary costs. Federation of Medical Boards of the United States, Inc. *Guide*, Section IX. The federation also recommends authority to impose stipulations, limitations, and conditions on the disciplined physician's scope of practice. The federation also recommends that various remedies be available to state licensure boards in disciplinary proceedings. Ibid., Section X.

78. See R. Walzer and S. Miltimore. 1993. "Mandated Supervision, Monitoring and Therapy of Disciplined Health Care Professionals." *Journal of Legal Medicine* 14: 565, 570–73.

79. See Jost, "Oversight of the Quality of Medical Care," 863; Grand and Marti, *Physicians' Licensure*, 173–74.

80. Grad and Marti, *Physicians' Licensure*, 175–76.

81. See S. Wolfe. 1992. "Public Access to Discipline Data." *Federation Bulletin* (December): 219.

82. See Davis and Pierce. *Administrative Law*, § 11.1, at 173; Schwartz, *Administrative Law*, § 8.1, at 470.

83. Furrow et al., *Health Law*, 1, § 3-19, at 113; Morris, *Revocation*, § 6-1, at 123; Grad and Marti, *Physicians' Licensure*, 177.

84. See, e.g., *Ortwein v. Schwab*, 410 U.S. 656 (1973). See Davis and Pierce, *Administrative Law*, § 11.1, at 178.

85. Furrow et al., *Health Law*, 1, §§ 3-23–3-24, at 121–24; Morris, *Revocation*, § 6-1, at 125; Grad and Marti, *Physicians' Licensure*, 7.

86. See Schwartz, *Administrative Law*, § 10.12, at 647–48; Davis and Pierce, *Administrative Law*, § 11.1, at 173.

87. See Furrow et al., *Health Law*, 1, §§ 3-23–3-24, at 121–24; Morris, *Revocation*, § 6-1, at 124; Grad and Marti, *Physicians' Licensure*, 178.

88. Model State Administrative Procedure Act, 1981 Act (U.L.A.) § 5-106; Model State Administrative Procedure Act, 1961 Act (U.L.A.) § 7, at 15.

89. Federation of State Medical Boards of the United States, Inc. *Guide*, Section X.

90. Model State Administrative Procedure Act, 1981 Act (U.L.A.) § 5-116; Model State Administrative Procedure Act, 1961 Act (U.L.A.) § 15(g).

91. 5 U.S.C. § 706(b) (1994).

92. See, e.g., *Bevacqua v. Sobol* 176 A.D.2d 1 (N.Y. App. Div. 1992); *Montalvo v. Mississippi State Board of Medical Licensure* 671 So.2d 53 (Miss. 1996). See Schwartz, *Administrative Law*, § 10.7, at 637–40.

93. See, e.g., *Bryce v. Board of Medical Quality Assurance*, 229 Cal. Rptr. 483 (Cal. App. 1986); *Arthur v. District of Columbia Nurses' Examining Board*, 459 A.2d 141 (D.C. 1983).

94. See, e.g., *Bettencourt v. Board of Registration*, 558 N.E.2d 928 (Mass. 1990); *Franz v. Board of Medical Quality Assurance*, 181 Cal. Rptr. 732 (Cal. 1982); *Gingo v.*

State Medical Board, 564 N.E.2d 1096 (Ohio App. 1989); *Abraham v. Ambach*, 522 N.Y.S.2d 318 (App. Div. 1987); *Garad v. State Board* 747 S.W.2d 726 (Mo. App. 1988). See Furrow et al., § 3–19, at 113; Morris, *Revocation*, § 6-1, at 129–30.

95. See Morris, *Revocation*, § 6-1, at 128; Grad and Marti, *Physicians' Licensure*, 178.

96. Citizen Advocacy Center. 1992. *A Resource Guide for Medical Boards Seeking to Limit Judicial Stays of Board Disciplinary Orders*. Washington, DC: AARP, 4–6.

97. See, e.g., *Commission on Medical Discipline v. Stillman*, 435 A.2d 747 (Md. 1981); *Board of Registration and Examination v. Stidd*, 377 N.E.2d 896 (Ind. App. 1978); *Flynn v. Board of Registration in Optometry*, 67 N.E.2d 846 (Mass. 1945). See Morris, *Revocation*, § 6-4, at 149–53.

98. Ibid., Citizen Advocacy Center, *Judicial Stays of Board Disciplinary Orders*, 4–6.

99. Ibid.

100. Schwartz, *Administrative Law*, § 3-1, at 110.

101. Grad and Marti, *Physicians' Licensure*, 156–57.

102. Jost, "Consumers, Complaints, and Professional Discipline," 315.

103. Jost, "Oversight of the Quality of Medical Care," 863–65.

104. Ibid.

105. Ibid.

106. See OIG, *State Medical Boards*, 3; Jost, "Consumers, Complaints, and Professional Discipline," 315.

107. Federation of State Medical Boards of the United States, Inc. *Exchange*, 17.

108. Ibid.

109. Schwartz, *Administrative Law*, § 7.16, at 403.

110. Schwartz, *Administrative Law*, § 3.17, at 146–48.

111. Grad and Marti, *Physicians' Licensure*, 164.

112. Ibid.

113. Ibid., 166–68.

114. Ibid.

115. See, e.g., AARP, *Effective Physician Oversight*, 10; OIG, *State Medical Boards*, 17.

116. AARP, *Effective Physician Oversight*, 10.

117. See Advisory Committee on Public Disclosure of Physician Information to the Secretary of Consumer Affairs and Business Regulation. 1995. *Making Informed Choices about Doctors*. Boston, MA: Department of Consumer Affairs and Business Regulation.

118. D. R. Norton. 1995. *Special Study—The Health Regulatory System: A Report to the Arizona Legislature by the Auditor General*. Phoenix, AZ: Office of the Auditor General, 21.

119. OIG, *State Medical Boards*, 17.

120. Health Care Quality Improvement Act of 1986, Pub. L. No. 99-660, §§ 421-31, 100 Stat. 3784, 3788–92 (codified as amended at 42 U.S.C. § 42 U.S.C. § 11111 (1994)).

121. I. Van Tuninen, P. McCarthy, and S. Wolfe. 1991. *Questionable Doctors Disciplined by States or Federal Government: A Public Citizen Health Research Group Report*. Washington, DC: Public Citizens Research Group.

122. Grad and Marti, *Physicians' Licensure*, 167–68.

123. Grad and Marti, *Physicians' Licensure*, 167.

124. Federation of State Medical Boards of the United States, Inc. *Guide*, Section X.

125. 564 N.E.2d 1046 (N.Y. 1990).

126. Ibid., at 1049.

127. 177 W.Va. 316, 352 S.E.2d 66 (W.Va. 1986).

128. 352 S.E.2d at 71.

129. 191 W.Va. 15, 442 S.E.2d 712 (W.Va. 1994).

6

THE ROLE OF PROFESSIONAL
SELF-REGULATION

David Orentlicher[1]

I N DECIDING the role of self-regulation in professional regulation, society faces an inevitable tension between its dependence on professional expertise and its distrust of professional self-interest. Not surprisingly, society has developed several approaches to regulating the healthcare professions, relying on self-regulation to some extent, but also on external forms of regulation. Professional societies establish practice guidelines,[2] insurers employ utilization review,[3] and courts are available to hear charges of professional malpractice. The purpose of this chapter is not to determine which of these approaches is most valuable. There is undoubtedly a role for all of them, with the importance of each approach depending upon the specific practice at stake. Indeed, a combination of approaches will often make the most sense.

This chapter will make three important points. First, professional societies can play, and have played, an important role in establishing guidelines for healthcare practitioners. Second, merely setting standards is insufficient to shape professional behavior; the standards generally need to be supplemented by incentives or mandates to ensure compliance by practitioners. Third, professional societies are much more successful at setting standards than they are at ensuring acceptance and implementation of the standards. The incentives or mandates necessary for compliance with standards of practice have generally come from outside the professions.

In developing these points, the chapter will refer to empirical studies of efforts to regulate physician behavior, as well as the author's own experience in trying to shape physician behavior through the drafting of ethical guidelines as director of the division of medical ethics at the AMA from 1989 to 1995. But before getting into specific examples, the discussion will focus on why it is important for healthcare professions to have some responsibility for establishing guidelines on matters of practice.

Professional Responsibility

There are several reasons why healthcare professions ought to have an important role in the setting of standards of practice.

Professional Autonomy

In the past two or three decades, patient autonomy has become the dominant ethical principle in healthcare.[4] Patient self-determination has replaced beneficence by the healthcare provider as the fundamental value in medical decision making.[5] Indeed, as David Blake has observed, when courts are faced with a patient's request to discontinue life-sustaining treatment, they almost uniformly give lip service to the state's interests in continuing treatment and in upholding the ethical integrity of medicine, and they ultimately defer to the patient's preferences.[6] In the liberal democratic state, in which there seldom is consensus on what is good, individuals must be given considerable freedom from externally imposed moral values. It is incumbent upon the state to maintain moral neutrality and permit individuals to define their own sense of morality, as long as there is no infringement on the freedom of fellow citizens.[7]

Healthcare providers also have a strong need for personal autonomy. Society respects individual dignity by permitting people to have control over essential aspects of their lives, and for most people, professional expression is a critical element of personhood. As Robert Gordon has noted, control over the working environment is a basic "precondition to the realization of [a] free, authentic personality."[8] To be sure, within the liberal state there may be subcommunities of persons who share a common moral view,[9] and healthcare providers may each therefore agree to be bound by a professional code of ethics. Nevertheless, principles of personal self-expression indicate that it is still for the profession, rather than the state, to develop a professional code.

Patients also benefit from the autonomy of healthcare providers. The healthcare professions will not attract talented individuals if practitioners are not given the opportunity for self-regulation. Currently, in explaining an increasing disenchantment with their professional lives, physicians identify loss of autonomy as one of the most important problems.[10] Doctors express substantial concern about mounting paperwork, heavy-handed utilization review, and greater government regulations—the so-called "hassle factor."[11] Such a reaction is predictable. As studies have demonstrated, when individuals exercise more control over decision making in their workplace, they experience greater satisfaction and are more productive in their employment.[12]

Reliability

Professional self-regulation in healthcare is important because laypeople do not have sufficient expertise to set standards for medical practice. With their training and experience, for example, physicians are much better equipped than other persons to establish practice guidelines for the diagnosis of illness and its medical or surgical treatment.[13] Similarly, nurses are in the best position to develop guidelines for the delivery of nursing care, and pharmacists are in the best position to develop guidelines for pharmacy services. Accordingly, courts have traditionally relied on the healthcare professions to establish standards for determining whether their members are practicing competently.[14]

Acceptability

Ethical guidelines will be more readily accepted by healthcare providers if they are developed internally rather than if they are imposed by external bodies, particularly external bodies with a poor record of self-regulation. For example, it is easy for physicians to dismiss calls by Congress for stricter rules on conflicts of interest in medicine when members of Congress routinely accept contributions from businesses that are affected by potential legislation. When healthcare providers assume responsibility for standard setting, they are more likely to feel invested in the process and to feel that the standards take due account of their concerns. Indeed, the approach of CQI has succeeded in improving healthcare services because it depends in part on healthcare providers helping to shape the processes by which they provide care to patients.[15]

The public also appears to hold more trust in the healthcare professions than in other bodies when it comes to setting ethical standards. In polls taken over the past fifteen years, 50 to 60 percent of those surveyed gave a "high" or "very high" rating to physicians on both honesty and ethical standards.[16] In contrast, only 10 to 25 percent of the respondents rated members of Congress as having "high" or "very high" ethical standards and only 10 to 20 percent of respondents gave a "high" or "very high" rating to state or local office-holders.[17] Similarly, on the question of whom the public trusts for proposing fair and workable health policies, 71 percent of those surveyed trusted organized medicine "some" or "a great deal," while only 40 percent trusted the federal government "some" or "a great deal."[18]

Independence from Political Processes

While professional self-regulation has inherent conflicts of interest and may be compromised by political pressures, too great a reliance on government regulation risks even greater politicization of the standard-setting process. Examples from recent presidential administrations are illustrative. Political considerations prevented the Reagan and Bush Administrations from even convening a federal ethics commission, despite congressional authorization,[19] and delayed for more than four years the implementation of recommendations by a federal advisory panel on fetal tissue transplantation.[20] When issues are settled in the political arena, the outcome tends to reflect compromises and balances of raw power rather than the principled resolution of conflicting moral considerations.

In some cases, independent government commissions can be used to insulate standard setters from political influences. Difficult political questions, like the closing of military bases, are often resolved by the establishment of "blue-ribbon" panels that make recommendations to Congress after careful study.[21] However, the recent politicization of Supreme Court appointments reflects how difficult it is to maintain the independence and integrity of government bodies that have a continuing responsibility.[22]

Due Process

According to principles of due process, healthcare providers ought to have the opportunity to resolve problems within the profession before other groups jump in with externally developed mandates. Due process recognizes that, in ensuring a just outcome, the mechanism for achieving a result is as important as the result itself.[23] Indeed, the tradition of oral argument in appellate litigation is important not so much because it affects the court's decision but because oral argument assures the litigants that they themselves have been heard.[24] As part of due process, courts generally do not review administrative agency decisions until challenges have been taken through administrative appeal (i.e., administrative remedies have been exhausted).[25] Requiring the exhaustion of administrative remedies provides administrative agencies the opportunity to correct their mistakes before courts step in.[26] Just as administrative agencies are given a chance to correct errors internally, so should the healthcare professions be permitted to correct problems through self-regulation before others step in with their own approaches.

Case Studies

Giving theoretical arguments to justify professional self-regulation is only part of the story. The question remains as to whether professional self-regulation actually works. Can the healthcare professions engage in meaningful self-regulation, or is this just a matter of letting foxes guard the chicken coop? The medical profession's experience with standard setting suggests the following conclusion: professional regulation can have a substantial effect on the behavior of practitioners, but professional guidelines alone are generally insufficient to change professional behavior. The guidelines must be combined with incentives or mandates to ensure compliance. Moreover, these incentives and mandates generally come from outside the profession.

Two sources of data can provide information on the effectiveness of professional standards: the effect of the AMA's guidelines on ethical questions and the effect of professional guidelines for therapeutic procedures such as guidelines that indicate when cesarean sections and coronary artery bypass surgery should be performed. While the experience with both types of guidelines is relevant, an assessment of the AMA's ethical guidelines must rely in part on anecdotal data; well-controlled studies of their effect do not exist. These are, on the other hand, many studies of the effect of professional guidelines on therapeutic procedures.

The AMA's Ethical Guidelines

The AMA's Council on Ethical and Judicial Affairs issues a *Code of Medical Ethics*[27] for physicians. Physicians who violate the AMA's code are subject to discipline by the AMA, and by their county and state medical societies.[28] A number of specialty societies, including the American Academy of Family Physicians and the American Psychiatric Association, have adopted the AMA's code and hold their members accountable for violations.[29] In some states, the medical licensing statute expressly considers violations of the AMA's code as grounds for discipline.[30] Apparently, state licensing boards generally view the AMA's code as probative, though not dispositive, evidence of the expected standard of conduct when deciding whether a physician has committed professional misconduct.[31]

Drawing on the author's six-and-one-half years at the AMA, the chapter will discuss an example of successful self-regulation and an example of unsuccessful self-regulation and suggest why the two efforts had different results.

Gifts to Physicians from Industry

During the 1980s, there was increasing concern in the medical profession about gifts to physicians from pharmaceutical and other companies.[32] Commentators were troubled both by the magnitude and the kinds of industry gift giving.[33] The Senate Labor and Human Resources Committee developed data on magnitude, which tracked expenditures by eighteen large pharmaceutical companies on gifts to physicians between 1975 and 1988.[34] Over that period, after taking inflation into account, gift expenditures nearly quintupled.[35] There also appeared to be a greater tendency for companies to give gifts particularly likely to influence the treatment decisions of physicians. Gift giving extended well beyond pens, mugs, and grants for educational programs to all-expense-paid weekend trips at lavish resorts for physicians and their spouses,[36] frequent prescriber programs offering free airline tickets for every fifty prescriptions,[37] and "studies" that paid physicians hundreds of dollars if they prescribed expensive antibiotics and collected data that were essentially demographic in nature.[38]

By 1990, guidelines on gift giving had been issued by a number of professional societies, including the American College of Physicians,[39] the American College of Cardiology,[40] and England's Royal College of Physicians.[41] However, there was little evidence of change in industry gift-giving practices. While praiseworthy, the guidelines lacked specificity. For example, physicians were admonished to decline gifts that they were not willing to have "generally known" to others.[42] This vagueness made it difficult to charge anyone with violations of these guidelines.

Following nearly a year of deliberations, the AMA issued its own guidelines on gift giving in December 1990.[43] The guidelines explicitly prohibit cash payments, subsidies for the travel expenses of physicians attending conferences, gifts tied to prescribing practices, and any gift not related to patient care.[44] In addition, the guidelines limit the magnitude of individual gifts and require that grants to defray registration fees for educational conferences be given directly to conference sponsors and not to physicians.[45]

Ordinarily, it is difficult to measure the effect of ethical guidelines. It is not always certain whether ethical guidelines result in behavioral changes. Even when changes are detected, it is often not clear whether the changes reflect the ethical guidelines or other contemporaneous influences. For example, if there is an increase in services provided to the poor after the issuance of a guideline calling on physicians to care for the indigent, the increase may be the result of the ethical guideline or, perhaps, the result of a coincidental rise in Medicaid reimbursement rates.

With the AMA gift-giving guidelines, however, the effect was immediate and substantial. Companies canceled educational and promotional conferences that were not strong enough to attract physicians willing to pay their own travel expenses, and promotional dinners where physicians received a free meal and a $100 payment were also abandoned.[46] The AMA received calls from travel agencies complaining about the effect of the gift-giving guidelines on their businesses, and physicians reported that lavish evening receptions were disappearing at major medical meetings. In this case, the ethical guidelines changed physician behavior dramatically and meaningfully.

Why were these guidelines so successful? First, the pharmaceutical industry incorporated the guidelines into its ethics code for marketing practices.[47] As a result, the success of the guidelines was not solely dependent on the willingness of physicians to adhere to their ethical responsibilities. After implementation, drug companies generally stopped offering inappropriate gifts; thus physicians were not in a position to accept them. In fact, the industry probably did not fight the guidelines too vigorously because, in some ways, companies welcomed the restrictions. To a certain extent, gifts are given because of physician demand,[48] and once one company accedes to such demands, other companies must follow in order to remain competitive. Similarly, one company may initiate gift giving as a marketing strategy and other companies, for competitive reasons, feel compelled to match the strategy. A prohibition on gift giving levels the playing field for members of the industry, having the same effect as an agreement by the companies that they would not try to compete with each other through gift giving.[49]

Second, while there are more than one hundred drug companies, a small number of large companies dominate the market.[50] Consequently, in order to ensure that the guidelines achieved their purpose, it was necessary to achieve compliance from only a few major companies. Moreover, with the focus on just the dominant players in the industry, policing the guidelines became much easier as well.

Third, detection of violations is relatively easy. Gift giving occurs openly, and companies usually offer the same gift to hundreds, if not thousands of physicians. Physicians who support the guidelines as well as competitors of the gift-giving company are likely to be aware of violations and report them to the AMA. Indeed, in the months following the implementation of the guidelines, the AMA's attention was drawn to a number of apparent violations.[51]

Fourth, concern about government regulation gave both physicians and industry a strong incentive to follow the AMA's guidelines. Immediately following the issuance of the guidelines, Senator Edward Kennedy convened hearings on the pharmaceutical industry's gift-giving practices.[52] After the hearings, he indicated that he would refrain from taking any legislative or regulatory action if the AMA's guidelines eliminated abusive gift-giving practices.[53] The increased attention to gift-giving practices encouraged the Office of the Inspector General at the U.S. Department of Health and Human Services to scrutinize pharmaceutical gifts more closely and to begin pursuing investigations of some of the more egregious practices to determine whether they violated federal statutes prohibiting kickbacks for drugs whose costs are reimbursed by Medicare or Medicaid.[54]

Fifth, the guidelines draw a number of "bright line" rules, establishing clear distinctions between permissible and impermissible conduct.[55] The pharmaceutical industry had previously adopted the American College of Physician's guidelines on gift-giving practices, but, because those guidelines essentially enunciated general principles, industry had a good deal of freedom in interpreting them.[56]

In short, the AMA gift-giving guidelines probably succeeded because the rules were clear,[57] because they actually served the interests of one of the parties affected, because there was a credible threat of enforcement in the form of greater government oversight, and because violations could be detected with relative ease.

Treatment of HIV-Infected Patients

There has apparently been less success with the AMA's ethical guideline on the duty of physicians to treat patients with HIV infection. In December 1987, the AMA's Council on Ethical and Judicial Affairs issued a guideline stating that physicians may not refuse to treat patients on account of their HIV infection.[58] Since then, however, studies suggest that a substantial number of physicians have not followed the guideline.[59] In an August 1990 random national sample of primary care physicians, 50 percent of the physicians surveyed stated that, if given a choice, they would not work with AIDS patients, and 48 percent stated that they preferred to refer patients with HIV infection to other physicians.[60] Similarly, in a survey of one thousand surgeons, more than 90 percent expressed support for a policy of refusing to operate on patients with HIV infection.[61] Since these surveys report attitudes rather than actual practices, it is possible that the surveyed physicians overcame their unwillingness to treat patients with HIV infection and hewed to their ethical responsibilities. Indeed, a 1986 survey of orthopedic surgeons suggested that, while more than two-thirds of orthopedists believed that a surgeon could ethically refuse to operate on a patient with HIV infection, 90 percent of the orthopedists who had an opportunity to operate on infected patients had done so on at least one patient with HIV infection.[62]

Several other studies, however, indicate that actual practices deviate from the ethical duty to treat. In a survey of Los Angeles County primary care physicians in late 1990, researchers found that 48 percent of the physicians surveyed either had refused or would refuse to accept HIV-infected patients into their practice.[63] Similarly, in a June 1990 survey of North Carolina physicians, 40 percent reported that they either refused to treat HIV-infected patients or referred the patients elsewhere.[64] In a 1989 survey of resident physicians, 39 percent of those surveyed in the United States reported that at least one of their HIV-infected patients had been refused care by a surgeon.[65] Finally, a 1989 national survey of 560 randomly selected hospitals found that 20 percent of these hospitals had experienced at least one case of a staff member refusing to treat a patient with HIV infection; 25 percent of the hospitals immediately transferred HIV-infected patients to other hospitals.[66]

Why has there apparently been less success with the guideline on the duty to treat patients with HIV infection than with the guideline on gifts from industry? A number of possible explanations come to mind. First, there are strong personal incentives to ignore the obligation to provide treatment. Physicians, particularly surgeons, are concerned that they will become infected from HIV patients while treating them.[67] While the perceived risk may be greater than the actual risk, it is perceptions that drive behavior. Physicians may also be discouraged from treating HIV-infected patients because of the psychological burdens of providing care. That is, because persons with AIDS experience severe and debilitating illness, caring for HIV-infected patients is often time-consuming and emotionally draining.

Second, it is easy to camouflage violations of the obligation to treat. Physicians who do not want to treat a patient with HIV infection can simply tell the patient that they are not taking any new patients, or that they accept patients only through a referral.[68]

These two examples of ethics guidelines suggest two important points. First, the medical profession is capable of devising meaningful and responsible guidelines on ethical matters, even when guidelines require conduct that might not be in the physician's own personal interest. Second, the profession is less successful when it comes to ensuring that guidelines are followed. Consequently, guidelines will probably not be adopted in practice unless there is some incentive or mandate that comes from outside the profession. As discussed in the next section, these two lessons can also be derived from the medical profession's experience with practice guidelines.

Practice Guidelines

To ensure that physician practices are consistent with quality medical care, professional societies have developed standards of practice for a wide range of clinical situations. The American Academy of Pediatrics has published schedules for childhood vaccinations;[69] the American College of Cardiology has issued guidelines for exercise testing,[70] coronary artery bypass surgery,[71] and pacemaker implantation;[72] and the American Society of Anesthesiologists has established standards for anesthetic monitoring during surgery.[73] Panels of experts developed these guidelines, based on published data and their own clinical experience.[74]

In general, studies have shown that simply developing and disseminating practice guidelines are not sufficient to change physician behavior, even when there is widespread knowledge among physicians about the guidelines. Additional measures are generally needed to ensure that the guidelines are actually followed. Moreover, these additional measures have generally come from outside the profession.

For example, despite the efforts of professional societies to reduce the rate of cesarean sections, the rate has remained high in both the United States and Canada.[75] After Canada's Society of Obstetricians and Gynecologists issued its practice guidelines for cesarean sections, roughly 90 percent of obstetricians surveyed reported that they knew about the guidelines, and more than 80 percent reported that they agreed with the guidelines.[76] Yet two years after the release of the guidelines, there was only a small decrease in the cesarean section rate.[77] Indeed, if that small a decline were multiplied over time, it would take more than thirty years for Canada's cesarean section rate to reach the medically desirable level.[78]

Similar results were found in a study of practice guidelines issued by the National Institutes of Health (NIH). Between 1977 and 1986, the NIH developed guidelines on sixty different practice questions.[79] In a study of the effect of four of those guidelines (two that applied to treatment of breast cancer, one that applied to cesarean sections, and one that applied to coronary artery bypass surgery), researchers found that the guidelines were largely unsuccessful in changing physician behavior.[80]

The failure of information alone to change physician behavior is not surprising. Sociological studies on the diffusion of innovation in medicine, in agriculture, and in other settings have come to the same conclusion: knowledge about and availability of an innovation are almost never adequate by themselves to cause adoption of the innovation.[81]

There are a number of reasons why physician behavior does not change by the mere dissemination of practice guidelines. Some studies suggest that physicians may be influenced more by their own clinical experiences than by studies in the literature or recommendations of experts.[82] Physicians may also resist practice guidelines as an unwarranted intrusion on their decision-making authority.[83] Indeed, some theoretical inquiries suggest that personal independence is a fundamental element of professionalism in the United States.[84]

Other factors underlying the resistance to change include personal interests and patient preferences. For example, in the case of cesarean sections, physicians may continue performing the procedure unnecessarily because they believe doing so will reduce their risk of malpractice liability—a jury might mistakenly attribute a newborn's prelabor injury to the use of vaginal delivery. Physicians may also be responding to other financial and personal incentives to perform cesarean sections, primarily that cesarean sections are more remunerative and require less time than vaginal deliveries.[85] Finally, physicians may be acceding to their patients' requests for cesarean sections (which may stem from a patient's wish to avoid a painful and prolonged delivery).[86]

The failure of practice guidelines to change behavior cannot be attributed simply to the inability of physicians to modify well-entrenched practices. There are a number of cases in which the medical profession has rapidly adapted to medical innovations, even without the issuance of practice guidelines. For example, within five years of its introduction in the United States, laparoscopic cholecystectomy had replaced more traditional surgical methods in roughly 80 percent of operations to remove the gallbladder.[87] This rapid adoption of a new procedure is particularly striking given the unavailability of any rigorous studies comparing the two procedures,[88] and the fact that laparoscopic surgery involves techniques very different from those used in more traditional forms of surgery.[89]

In some cases, practice guidelines have been successful in changing physician behavior. While the successes have come in different ways, the different mechanisms for change have generally come from outside the profession. For example, the successful implementation of standards for anesthetic monitoring was a result of a combination of mandates from both hospitals and licensing boards for their use,[90] and reductions in malpractice premiums that were conditioned on their use.[91]

Strict regulatory oversight has been cited as a mechanism for ensuring adherence to practice guidelines in other settings. In a study of coronary artery bypass surgery in New York State, researchers found a very low rate of inappropriate operations.[92] The authors of the study attributed the findings to the state government's careful regulation of bypass surgery, including the requirement that hospitals satisfy high standards of quality before they are certified or recertified as centers for open-heart surgery.[93] Similar results have been achieved by federal regulatory oversight. After the federal government imposed strict guidelines for the use of antipsychotic drugs in nursing homes, researchers found that there was a substantial decrease in antipsychotic drug use in Tennessee nursing homes.[94]

Reimbursement policies of healthcare insurers have also been important in ensuring adherence to practice guidelines. Before the issuance of guidelines on cardiac pacemaker implantation, data suggested that at least 20 percent of pacemakers were not warranted.[95] Following the issuance of the guidelines, there was a 28 percent decline in the use of pacemakers in Medicare patients.[96] The decline probably reflected the use of the pacemaker guidelines by the Medicare system in deciding when to cover pacemaker implantations.[97] Tying reimbursement to adherence to practice guidelines is an obvious method for achieving physician adoption of practice guidelines. Physicians are not very likely to perform procedures for which they are not compensated.

Indeed, the interesting question is why reimbursement has not been predicated more frequently on physician adherence to practice guidelines. For the most part, the answer probably lies in the fact that most practice guidelines have been developed relatively recently and are available for only a small percentage of medical decisions. In addition, as indicated above, there is a good deal of resistance by the medical profession to the imposition of practice guidelines. When Blue Cross and Blue Shield of Illinois disclosed its plan to require physicians in its managed care networks to follow practice guidelines, the AMA criticized the plan as an unwarranted intrusion on professional judgment by an insurance company.[98] Healthcare insurers may have resisted using their reimbursement policies to impose practice guidelines in the belief that the benefits of using practice guidelines did not outweigh the costs of antagonizing physicians.

There is one basis for adoption of practice guidelines that seems to come from within the medical profession. In several cases, such as the use of antibiotics or cesarean sections, practice guidelines have been adopted by physicians when local "opinion leaders" (physicians whose opinions tend to be followed by other physicians in their community) have adopted the guidelines and encouraged their colleagues to do so as well.[99] The phenomenon of opinion leadership is widely recognized and studied in the marketing and sociological literature.[100] Purveyors of consumer products have long known that, while media advertising is useful for making people aware of a new item, consumers often turn to influential friends and acquaintances for guidance when deciding whether to try the item.[101] The importance of opinion leadership for physicians was illustrated in a major study dealing with the adoption of a new prescription drug in four midwestern towns in the 1950s. Researchers found that the most important factor in explaining how rapidly a physician adopted the drug was whether the physician was well integrated into professional and social networks with other physicians.[102] Physicians who were professionally and socially isolated tended to be much slower to incorporate the drug into their practice.[103]

While opinion leadership helps us understand the adoption of practice guidelines, it does not provide a full explanation of the process of adoption. Opinion leadership explains how a new practice spreads through the profession. However, it does not explain how the process of adoption begins. We still are left with mechanisms for ensuring adoption of practice guidelines that come from outside the profession. The mere issuance of guidelines by professional societies rarely suffices to change physician behavior. Rather, mandates or financial incentives are typically needed.

The Need for External Incentives or Mandates

An important question is why physicians seem to be much more successful at creating standards than ensuring compliance with those standards. Why has this been the case? First, there is a natural reluctance to engage in enforcement when the discipline is meted out to colleagues. Members of a commission investigating police corruption in New York City came to a similar conclusion: police corruption exists, despite such periodic investigatory commissions, because police are reluctant to clamp down when they discover corruption in the ranks.[104] Physicians, like other professionals engaged in self-regulation, can readily sympathize with the ethical lapses of their peers because it is easy to imagine themselves making similar errors. Moreover, medicine has always been an unusually collegial profession. The Hippocratic oath[105] instructs physicians to give special preference to the sons of their colleagues, and fealty to the profession is considered as important in the oath as devotion to patients.

Self-enforcement is also weak because it is poorly funded. Physicians who serve on the disciplinary committees of their professional bodies do so without compensation. In addition, there is little money available for staff, and the committees have no subpoena authority. Consequently, few cases can be pursued, and rigorous investigations are not possible. Moreover, even when cases are prosecuted, there are substantial financial risks to the professional society. Physicians who are disciplined often challenge their sanction through time-consuming and costly litigation. Indeed, the legal fees for defending a case can deplete much of a small medical society's annual budget. Antitrust liability is of particular concern with its potential for treble damage and attorneys' fee awards.[106] As the U.S. Congress found when it enacted the Health Care Quality Improvement Act of 1986[107] to provide physicians some protection against retaliatory lawsuits, the threat of liability "unreasonably discourages physicians from participating in effective professional peer review."[108]

Conclusion

As policymakers consider how to regulate the practices of healthcare providers, they should recognize the important differences between *establishing* and *enforcing* professional guidelines. The medical profession's experience with ethics guidelines and practice guidelines indicates that society may be able to rely on the healthcare professions to develop responsible standards. In addition, principles of change theory suggest that healthcare providers will be more receptive to restrictions on their autonomy if they are involved in the process of developing the restrictions.[109] However, on the issue of enforcement, reliable mechanisms have come from outside the profession, generally in the form of regulatory mandates or reimbursement policies.

Two important caveats are in order. First, the experiences of the medical profession may not be representative of other healthcare professions. Second, it is likely that the establishment and enforcement of guidelines are related rather than independent endeavors. Specifically, the willingness of the healthcare professions to enact responsible guidelines might diminish if robust enforcement mechanisms were in place. It may be that tough guidelines can be adopted precisely because there often is little risk that they will be enforced. On the other hand, the alternative of having outside groups establish the guidelines might provide sufficient incentive for the professions to continue developing rigorous ethical standards even under a system of regular, reliable enforcement. How all this would play out is indeterminate; whether enhanced enforcement would diminish the zeal of professional standard setting is an empirical question that can be resolved only by monitoring the regulatory process and measuring the effect of greater enforcement activities.

Notes

1. This chapter is adapted from an article originally published as D. Orentlicher. 1994. "The Influence of a Professional Organization on Physician Behavior." *Albany Law Review* 57 (3): 583, with permission of the *Albany Law Review*.

2. Committee on Pacemaker Implantation, American College of Cardiology/American Heart Association Task Force on Assessment of Diagnostic and Therapeutic Cardiovascular Procedures. 1991. "Guidelines for Implantation of Cardiac Pacemakers and Antiarrhythmia Devices." *Journal of the American College of Cardiology* 18 (1): 1.

3. M. S. Barr and T. R. Marmor. 1992. "Making Sense of the National Health Insurance Reform Debate." *Yale Law and Policy Review* 10 (2): 228.

4. T. L. Beauchamp and J. F. Childress. 1989. *Principles of Biomedical Ethics*, 3rd edit. New York: Oxford University Press, 67–113.

5. Ibid., 210.

6. D. C. Blake. 1989. "State Interests in Terminating Medical Treatment." *Hastings Center Report* 19 (3): 5.

7. H. T. Engelhardt, Jr. 1986. *The Foundations of Bioethics*. New York: Oxford University Press, 17–56.

8. R. W. Gordon. 1989. "The Independence of Lawyers." *Boston University Law Review* 68 (1): 1, 9.

9. Engelhardt, *Foundations*, 49–56.

10. A. M. Epstein. 1993. "Changes in the Delivery of Care under Comprehensive Health Care Reform." *New England Journal of Medicine* 329 (22): 1672, 1673.

11. Ibid.

12. R. J. Bullock. 1984. *Improving Job Satisfaction*. New York: Pergamon Press, 4–5; K. I. Miller and P. R. Monge. "Participation, Satisfaction, and Productivity: A Meta-Analytic Review." *Academic Management Journal* 29 (4): 727.

13. W. P. Keeton, D. B. Dobbs, R. E. Keeton, and D. G. Owen (eds.). 1984. *Prosser and Keeton on the Law of Torts*, 5th edit. St. Paul, MN: West Publishing Co., 189.

14. Ibid., 185–89.

15. D. M. Berwick. 1989. "Continuous Improvement as an Ideal in Health Care." *New England Journal of Medicine* 320 (1): 53.

16. L. McAneny. 1993. "Honesty and Ethics Poll: Pharmacists Retain Wide Lead as Most Honorable Profession." *Los Angeles Times Syndicate*, 29 July.

17. Ibid.

18. L. K. Harvey. 1991. *AMA Survey of Public Opinion on Health Care Issues*. Chicago: American Medical Association, 18.

19. Office of Technology Assessment, U.S. Congress. 1993. *Biomedical Ethics in U.S. Public Policy*. Washington, DC: U.S. Government Printing Office.

20. Ibid., 9.

21. E. Schmitt. 1993. "A Mission Accomplished." *New York Times*, 29 June, A10.

22. W. G. Ross. 1994. "The Supreme Court Appointment Process: A Search for a Synthesis." *Albany Law Review* 57 (4): 993.

23. J. E. Nowak and R. D. Rotunda. 1991. *Constitutional Law*, 4th edit. St. Paul, MN:

West Publishing Co., 487.

24. R. L. Stern. 1989. *Appellate Practice in the United States*, 2nd edit. Washington, DC: Bureau of National Affairs, 365–70.

25. *Myers v. Bethlehem Shipbuilding Corporation*, 303 U.S. 41, 50-51 (1938).

26. K. C. Davis and R. J. Pierce, Jr. 1994. *Administrative Law Treatise*, 3rd edit. Boston: Little Brown and Co., 309.

27. Council on Ethical and Judicial Affairs. 1996. *Code of Medical Ethics: Current Opinions with Annotations*, 1996–97 edition. Chicago: American Medical Association.

28. Council, *Code of Medical Ethics*, 1, 142–43, 170–74.

29. American Academy of Family Physicians. 1993. *Bylaws*. Kansas City, MO: American Academy of Family Physicians, 6–7; American Psychiatric Association. 1989. *The Principles of Medical Ethics: With Annotations Especially Applicable to Psychiatry*. Washington, DC: American Psychiatric Association.

30. *Ohio Rev. Code Ann.* § 4731.22(B)(18) (Anderson Supp. 1995).

31. Telephone interview with Dorothy Harwood, Assistant Vice President for Administrative and Legislative Affairs, Federation of State Medical Boards of the United States, 3 Feb. 1994.

32. M. Chren, C. S. Landefeld, and T. H. Murray. 1989. "Doctors, Drug Companies, and Gifts." *Journal of the American Medical Association* 262 (24): 3448; S. E. Goldfinger. 1987. "A Matter of Influence." *New England Journal of Medicine* 316 (22): 1408; M. D. Rawlins. 1984. "Doctors and the Drug Makers." *Lancet* (Aug. 4): 276.

33. Council on Ethical and Judicial Affairs, American Medical Association. 1991. "Gifts to Physicians from Industry." *Journal of the American Medical Association* 265 (4): 501; J. Graves. 1987. "Frequent-Flyer Programs for Drug Prescribing." *New England Journal of Medicine* 317 (4): 252; T. Randall. 1991. "Kennedy Hearings Say No More Free Lunch—or Much Else—From Drug Firms." *Journal of the American Medical Association* 265 (4): 440.

34. Randall, "Kennedy Hearings," 440, 442.

35. Ibid., 442.

36. J. C. Nelson. 1990. "A Snorkel, a 5-Iron, and a Pen." *Journal of the American Medical Association* 264 (6): 742.

37. Graves, "Frequent-Flyer," 252.

38. Randall, "Kennedy Hearings," 440.

39. American College of Physicians. 1990. "Physicians and the Pharmaceutical Industry." *Annals of Internal Medicine* 112 (8): 624.

40. C. R. Conti, J. F. Williams, Jr., J. L. Anderson, H. A. Berman, R. M. Gunnar, G. P. Herman, F. W. Lyons, Jr., E. R. Passamani, P. R. Reid, M. E. Silverman, S. L. Weinberg, and L. Yerkes. 1990. "Task Force V: The Relation of Cardiovascular Specialists to Industry, Institutions and Organizations." *Journal of the American College of Cardiology* 16 (1): 30.

41. Royal College of Physicians. 1986. "The Relationship Between Physicians and the Pharmaceutical Industry." *Journal of the Royal College of Physicians of London* 20 (4): 235.

42. American College, "Physicians," 624; Conti et al., "Task Force V," 32; Royal

College, "The Relationship," 238.

43. Council, "Gifts to Physicians," 501.

44. Ibid.; Council, *Code of Medical Ethics*, 117–19.

45. Council, *Code of Medical Ethics*, 117–19; Council on Ethical and Judicial Affairs, American Medical Association. 1992. "Guidelines on Gifts to Physicians from Industry: An Update." *Food and Drug Law Journal* 47 (4): 445, 452.

46. T. Randall. 1991. "AMA, Pharmaceutical Association Form 'Solid Front' on Gift-Giving Guidelines." *Journal of the American Medical Association* 265 (18): 2304.

47. Ibid.

48. Royal College, "The Relationship," 237.

49. Such an agreement would, of course, be unlawful under antitrust law. 15 U.S.C. § 1 (1994). Agreeing to the AMA's code could also constitute a violation of antitrust law, but the risk of prosecution is very low.

50. A. J. Darnay. 1991. *Market Share Reporter: An Annual Compilation of Reported Market Share Data on Companies, Products, and Services.* Detroit, MI: Gale Research, 191–92.

51. Randall, "AMA, Pharmaceutical Association," 2304.

52. Randall, "Kennedy Hearings," 440.

53. Randall, "AMA, Pharmaceutical Association," 2305.

54. A. M. Kirschenbaum and B. N. Kuhlik. 1992. "Federal and State Laws Affecting Discounts, Rebates, and Other Marketing Practices for Drugs and Devices." *Food and Drug Law Journal* 47 (5): 533, 553–56.

55. Council, *Code of Medical Ethics*, 117–19.

56. Randall, "Kennedy Hearings," 442.

57. Clear guidelines were also a key factor in the success of a federal government regulation limiting the use of antipsychotic drugs in nursing homes. R. L. Kane and J. Garrard. 1994. "Changing Physician Prescribing Practices: Regulation vs. Education." *Journal of the American Medical Association* 271 (5): 393.

58. Council, *Code of Medical Ethics*, 157; Council on Ethical and Judicial Affairs. 1988. "Ethical Issues Involved in the Growing AIDS Crisis." *Journal of the American Medical Association* 259 (9): 1360.

59. ACLU AIDS Project. 1990. *Epidemic of Fear: A Survey of AIDS Discrimination in the 1980s and Policy Recommendations for the 1990s.* New York: American Civil Liberties Union, 78–80.

60. B. Gerbert, B. T. Maguire, T. Bleecker, T. J. Coates, and S. J. McPhee. 1991. "Primary Care Physicians and AIDS: Attitudinal and Structural Barriers to Care." *Journal of the American Medical Association* 266 (20): 2837, 2839.

61. ACLU, *Epidemic of Fear*, 80.

62. P. M. Arnow, L. A. Pottenger, C. B. Stocking, M. Siegler, and H. W. DeLeeuw. 1989. "Orthopedic Surgeons' Attitudes and Practices Concerning Treatment of Patients with HIV Infection." *Public Health Report* 104 (2): 121, 124, 127. Of course, it is possible that many of the 90 percent refused to treat the majority of HIV-infected patients who sought care from them.

63. C. E. Lewis and K. Montgomery. 1992. "Primary Care Physicians' Refusal to Care

for Patients Infected with the Human Immunodeficiency Virus." *Western Journal of Medicine* 156 (1): 36, 37.

64. M. Weinberger, C. J. Conover, G. P. Samsa, and S. M. Greenberg. 1992. "Physicians' Attitudes and Practices Regarding Treatment of HIV-Infected Patients." *Southern Medical Journal* 85 (7): 683, 685.

65. M. F. Shapiro, R. A. Hayward, D. Guillemot, and D. Jayle. 1992. "Residents' Experiences in, and Attitudes Toward, the Care of Persons with AIDS in Canada, France, and the United States." *Journal of the American Medical Association* 268 (4): 510, 512.

66. P. J. Hilts. 1990. "Many Hospitals Found to Ignore Rights of Patients in AIDS Testing." *New York Times*, 17 February, 1, 12.

67. Weinberger et al., "Physicians' Attitudes," 684.

68. M. H. Jackson and N. D. Hunter. 1992. "The Very Fabric of Health Care: The Duty of Health Care Providers to Treat People Infected with HIV." In *AIDS Agenda: Emerging Issues in Civil Rights*, edited by N. D. Hunter and W. B. Rubenstein, 123, 124. New York: New Press.

69. G. Peter (ed.). 1994. *1994 Red Book: Report of the Committee on Infectious Diseases* 23rd edit., 23–25. Elk Grove Village, IL: American Academy of Pediatrics.

70. Subcommittee on Exercise Testing, American College of Cardiology/American Heart Association Task Force on Assessment of Cardiovascular Procedures. 1986. "Guidelines for Exercise Testing." *Journal of the American College of Cardiology* 8 (3): 725.

71. Subcommittee on Coronary Artery Bypass Graft Surgery, American College of Cardiology/American Heart Association Task Force on Assessment of Diagnostic and Therapeutic Cardiovascular Procedures. 1991. "Guidelines and Indications for Coronary Artery Bypass Graft Surgery." *Journal of the American College of Cardiology* 17 (3): 543.

72. Committee on Pacemaker Implantation, "Guidelines for Implantation," 1.

73. E. C. Pierce, Jr. 1990. "The Development of Anesthesia Guidelines and Standards." *Quality Review Bulletin* 16 (2): 61.

74. J. T. Kelly and J. E. Swartwout. 1990. "Development of Practice Parameters by Physician Organizations." *Quality Review Bulletin* 16 (2): 54, 56.

75. U.S. Centers for Disease Control and Prevention. 1995. "Rates of Cesarean Delivery—United States, 1993." *Morbidity and Mortality Weekly Report* 44 (15): 303, 304.

76. J. Lomas, G. M. Anderson, K. Domnick-Pierre, E. Vayda, M. W. Enkin, and W. J. Hannah. 1989. "Do Practice Guidelines Guide Practice? The Effect of a Consensus Statement on the Practice of Physicians." *New England Journal of Medicine* 321 (19): 1306, 1308.

77. Ibid., 1310.

78. Ibid.

79. J. Kosecoff, D. E. Kanouse, W. H. Rogers, L. McCloskey, C. M. Winslow, and R. H. Brook. 1987. "Effects of the National Institutes of Health Consensus Development Program on Physician Practice." *Journal of the American Medical Association* 258 (19): 2708.

80. Ibid., 2712.

81. J. S. Coleman, E. Katz, and H. Menzel. 1966. *Medical Innovation: A Diffusion*

Study. Indianapolis, IN: Bobbs-Merrill Co., Inc., 25.

82. P. J. Greco and J. M. Eisenberg. 1993. "Changing Physicians' Practices." *New England Journal of Medicine* 329 (17): 1271; L. Pilote, R. J. Thomas, D. Dennis, P. Goins, N. Houston-Miller, H. Kraemer, C. Leong, W. E. Berger, III, H. Lew, and R. S. Heller. 1992. "Return to Work after Uncomplicated Myocardial Infarction: A Trial of Practice Guidelines in the Community." *Annals of Internal Medicine* 117 (5): 383, 388–89.

83. Greco and Eisenberg, "Changing Physicians' Practices," 1273.

84. B. J. Bledstein. 1976. *The Culture of Professionalism: The Middle Class and the Development of Higher Education in America*. New York: W. W. Norton & Co., Inc., 80, 91, 92.

85. Some healthcare insurers have responded to this incentive by reimbursing physicians the same amount for vaginal delivery as for cesarean delivery or by switching to capitated forms of reimbursement in which obstetricians would receive a flat fee for each patient regardless of the actual costs of care provided.

86. Lomas et al., "Do Practice Guidelines," 1310.

87. NIH Consensus Development Panel on Gallstones and Laparoscopic Cholecystectomy. 1993. "Gallstones and Laparoscopic Cholecystectomy." *Journal of the American Medical Association* 269 (8): 1018.

88. Ibid.

89. B. Gaster. 1993. "The Learning Curve." *Journal of the American Medical Association* 270 (11): 1280.

90. J. H. Eichhorn. 1989. "Prevention of Intraoperative Anesthesia Accidents and Related Severe Injury through Safety Monitoring." *Anesthesiology* 70 (4): 572; J. H. Eichhorn, J. B. Cooper, D. J. Cullen, W. R. Maier, J. H. Philip, and R. G. Seeman. 1986. "Standards for Patient Monitoring During Anesthesia at Harvard Medical School." *Journal of the American Medical Association* 256 (8): 1017.

91. Eichhorn, "Standards," 1017; Pierce, "The Development," 63.

92. L. L. Leape, L. H. Hilborne, R. E Park, S. J, Bernstein, C. J. Kamberg, M. Sherwood, and R. H. Brook. 1993. "The Appropriateness of Use of Coronary Artery Bypass Graft Surgery in New York State." *Journal of the American Medical Association* 269 (6): 753, 758.

93. Ibid., 760.

94. R. I. Shorr, R. L. Fought, and W. A. Ray. 1994. "Changes in Antipsychotic Drug Use in Nursing Homes During Implementation of the OBRA-87 Regulations." *Journal of the American Medical Association* 271 (5): 358.

95. A. M. Greenspan, H. R. Kay, B. C. Berger, R. M. Greenberg, A. J. Greenspon, and M. J. Gaughan. 1988. "Incidence of Unwarranted Implantation of Permanent Cardiac Pacemakers in a Large Medical Population." *New England Journal of Medicine* 318 (3): 158, 160.

96. J. B. Mitchell, G. Wedig, and J. Cromwell. 1989. "The Medicare Physician Fee Freeze: What Really Happened?" *Health Affairs* 8 (1): 21, 27.

97. Kelly and Swartwout, "Development," 54.

98. M. M. Millenson. 1993. "Blue Cross to Enforce Treatment Guidelines." *Chicago Tribune*, 10 November, 1.

99. D. E. Everitt, S. B. Soumerai, J. Avorn, H. Klapholz, and M. Wessels. 1990. "Changing Surgical Antimicrobial Prophylaxis Practices Through Education

Targeted at Senior Department Leaders." *Infection Control and Hospital Epidemiology* 11 (11): 578, 579; J. Lomas, M. Enkin, G. M. Anderson, W. J. Hannah, E. Vayda, and J. Singer. 1991. "Opinion Leaders vs. Audit and Feedback to Implement Practice Guidelines: Delivery after Previous Cesarean Section." *Journal of the American Medical Association* 265 (17): 2202, 2206.

100. K. K. Chan and S. Misra. 1990. "Characteristics of the Opinion Leader: A New Dimension." *Journal of Advertising* 19 (3): 53; D. Leonard-Barton. 1985. "Experts as Negative Opinion Leaders in the Diffusion of a Technological Innovation." *Journal of Consumer Research* 11 (4): 914.

101. Chan and Misra, "Characteristics," 53.

102. Coleman et al., *Medical Innovation*, 79–112.

103. Ibid.

104. J. P. Armao and L. U. Cornfeld. 1993. "Why Good Cops Turn Rotten." *New York Times*, 1 November, A19.

105. T. A. Mappes and J. S. Zembaty. 1991. *Biomedical Ethics*, 3rd edit. New York: McGraw-Hill: 53 (reprinting the Hippocratic oath).

106. W. J. Curran. 1987. "Medical Peer Review of Physician Competence and Performance: Legal Immunity and the Antitrust Laws." *New England Journal of Medicine* 316 (10): 597.

107. 42 U.S.C. §§ 11,101–11,152 (1994).

108. 42 U.S.C. § 11,101(4) (1994).

109. Greco and Eisenberg, "Changing Physicians' Practices," 1272.

PUBLIC LICENSURE, PRIVATE CERTIFICATION, AND CREDENTIALING OF MEDICAL PROFESSIONALS: AN ANTITRUST PERSPECTIVE

Thomas L. Greaney

MERICA'S EXTRAORDINARY reliance on private entities to regulate the quality of professional services has been widely observed. Deference to the judgments of medical professionals in matters regarding fitness for practice is traceable to the early nineteenth century when licensure was first instituted in several states and responsibility was delegated to medical societies.[1] This tradition persisted under the modern statutory framework that evolved around the turn of the century as public boards, dominated by organized medicine, assumed the licensing function and established self-regulation of medical education and specialty practice.[2] Although external controls in the form of governmental peer review and quality monitoring under Medicare and credentialing by hospitals developed later, even these processes were characterized by a significant degree of professional self-regulation.[3]

Professional dominion over providers' qualifications, the minimum standards for practice, terms of practice, conduct, and institutional arrangements seems largely to have been premised on market failure. It has long been assumed that inadequate and asymmetrically distributed information thwarted effective appraisals of the quality of health services by either consumers or their agents.[4] Moreover, certification and standards may in some circumstances constitute a "public good," underproduced in the marketplace, and demanding extramarket interventions to ensure that an "efficient" level of information is produced. Of course, the economist's traditional response to market failure of this sort is governmental intervention, not abdication to interested market participants. Nevertheless, perhaps owing to organized medicine's deft political maneuvering and opinion shaping, firm governmental control over the levers of quality was never established in the United States.[5] Thus, the notion that professionals should bear prime responsibility for making these determinations, and that they should do so free of governmental second-guessing, has been widely accepted throughout this century.

Despite today's increasing reliance on market-driven arrangements in healthcare delivery, there has been no wholesale rejection, either in public policy or in legal doctrine, of professional control over the instruments of quality monitoring. Profession-dominated institutions continue to control the qualifications for specialization,[6] the nature of medical education,[7] and other central aspects of medical services in the United States.[8] At the same time, however, quality monitors have proliferated. Spurred by the revolution in information processing and demands of the marketplace, networks, for-profit management companies, HMOs, employers, payors, and consultants all engage in quality control through credentialing, utilization review, and other management devices.[9]

Antitrust law, which limits the exercise of collective power over markets, plays a highly nuanced role in overseeing self-regulation by health professionals. Its role in supervising professional control over accrediting and licensing has been modest, at least when compared to its interventions involving health financing systems, networks, and mergers. As will be seen, a host of doctrines circumscribe application of antitrust law in this area. As a consequence, the core of "professionalism"—collective activities undertaken to certify professional competence, share scientific information, and promulgate standards—encounters virtually no hindrance from antitrust law. According to some observers, however, excessive solicitude of professional judgment on matters of credentials and quality standards may have helped reinforce the medical profession's hegemony over the market for information. In contrast to its hospitable tradition with regard to the core aspects of professionalism, antitrust has closely policed agreements of private associations that restrict members' actions or constrain the actions of others. Here one observes a policy of zero tolerance for collective action, even when justified by facially plausible professional concerns.

Antitrust Law and Healthcare Providers: Some Basic Tenets

Antitrust law examines the competitive consequences of private activities and is largely the product of judicial interpretation of broad legislative directives. It looks to curtail collaborations that constitute unreasonable restrictions on competition or that enable entities to exercise or obtain market power by improper means. Section One of the Sherman Act limits cooperative arrangements by prohibiting "every contract, combination . . . or conspiracy, in restraint of trade or commerce among the several states, or with foreign nations." Hence, only agreements (as contrasted with purely unilateral conduct) are prohibited. Over the years, courts have categorized conduct and developed presumptive rules for each category. Price fixing, boycotts that deny competitors access to markets or relationships needed to compete, and dividing markets are seen as particularly suspect activities.

Section Two of the Sherman Act prohibits unilateral conduct of parties that amounts to monopolization, an attempt to monopolize, or a conspiracy to monopolize. Courts have interpreted this section to require proof that the defendant possesses monopoly power in a relevant market and the "willful acquisition or maintenance of that power as distinguished from growth or development as a consequence of a superior product, business acumen, or historic accident."[10] The Clayton Act and the Federal Trade Commission Acts prohibit certain specific practices, while also granting the FTC power to condemn by rule making or adjudication "unfair methods of competition." The Clayton Act also condemns acquisitions (mergers, stock and asset acquisitions) that "may substantially lessen competition."

As mentioned, there is a substantial body of case law interpreting these statutes, particularly in the healthcare industry, which has been a frequent target of governmental and private antitrust actions.[11] Four principles of particular importance to evaluating actions relating to professional standards are discussed next.

Protection of Competition, Not Competitors

The often repeated maxim that the fundamental goal of antitrust law is to protect competition, not competitors[12] conveys an important principle underlying contemporary interpretations of the law. It recognizes that competitors will often be harmed or eliminated in the give-and-take of the marketplace and underscores that the proper focus of antitrust law is to punish only those who succeed by unfair means or the improper exercise of market power. Hence, injuries sustained by firms or individuals who have lost out because of the inadequacy of their service or even bad luck are not cognizable under antitrust law.

Quality of Care Justifications

The Supreme Court has flatly rejected the notion that certain practices, including those embodied in the ethical codes of a profession, should be excused because they promote safety, improve the quality of care, or promote other worthy goals.[13] Moreover, the status of medicine as a "learned profession" does not exempt the activities of practitioners. Despite language in one landmark Supreme Court decision, the professional status of physicians grants little, if any, special consideration under the antitrust laws.[14]

State Action

Antitrust law does not reach the anticompetitive actions of the states or their officers. In many instances, however, it is unclear whether private parties are acting under sufficient mandate from the state to protect their actions from antitrust challenge. A two-prong standard has emerged to test whether the activity of a private party will qualify for immunity under this so-called "state action doctrine": "First, the challenged restraint must be one clearly articulated and affirmatively expressed as state policy; second the policy must be 'actively supervised' by the state itself."[15] Where the actor is a state agency, local governmental entity, or special local governmental agency, only the first prong, the clear articulation test, need be met.

Soliciting Government Action

Competitors may solicit governmental action without violating the antitrust law, even though that action may restrain trade or create a monopoly. Under the *Noerr-Pennington* exemption, petitioning governmental entities (including the legislature, administrative agencies, and governmental payors) does not give rise to an antitrust cause of action despite any adverse competitive consequences that may flow from successful solicitation.[16] An exception to this exemption is for "sham" petitioning of the government, that is, using the governmental process as an anticompetitive tool, through such acts as defrauding the government, bringing objectively baseless litigation, or intentionally barring competitors access to governmental agencies.[17]

Governmental Activity: Licensure, Quality Control, and the Antitrust Laws

The ubiquitous and influential role played by private entities in the quality assurance process is evident both in the processes through which professionals are licensed and in the eligibility standards and quality review screens employed by governmental insurers. State licensing boards typically rely heavily on private consultants or associations for evaluations of practitioners' competence and other matters. Moreover, the relatively passive role of state licensing boards can be regarded as an implicit delegation of the principal quality assurance function to private decision makers in medical education, specialty boards, hospitals, networks, and payors. In other areas affecting quality of care, such as eligibility for participation in government health programs and institutional privileges, governmental entities explicitly delegate quality assurance functions to private entities.

As a general matter, the antitrust laws are aimed at the conduct of private parties, not those of governmental entities or their employees or agents. Based on the legislative intent of Congress in enacting the antitrust statutes and other legal doctrines, courts have held the federal government and its agents to be immune from antitrust suits. Hence, Medicare intermediaries acting in their official capacities are immune,[18] as are peer reviewers and others acting as agents of the federal government.[19]

Antitrust analyses of the activities of state governmental entities involved in licensure and peer review turn on the application of the state action doctrine. As discussed above, the Supreme Court has interpreted the Sherman Act not to proscribe state legislatures from supplanting competition with regulation. Thus, licensing activities undertaken by the state acting through its administrative agencies or those of local governments enjoy state action immunity, provided that the conduct is taken pursuant to a "clearly articulated and affirmatively expressed" state policy. The actions of private parties assisting the licensing body or soliciting it to act are shielded by this doctrine as well. (Moreover, *Noerr* immunity for governmental petitioning affords additional protection.)

Although the state action doctrine would seem to preclude most antitrust challenges to state licensure regulation, a number of cases have held that broad and imprecise delegations of authority to state regulators of professionals are inadequate to meet the clear articulation prong of the statute. A broad statutory grant to a board to "regulate" a profession or ensure high ethical standards does not necessarily grant the agency the power to ban advertising, mail-order business, or claims of superiority.[20] In addition, the provision of fraudulent facts to subvert the government's processes can, in theory, give rise to an antitrust violation, although these actions are extraordinarily difficult to sustain.[21] Nevertheless, no successful antitrust challenge has been brought against the core function of licensing professionals to practice a profession because that activity is clearly and affirmatively expressed in licensure statutes and would clearly qualify for immunity.

As to situations in which private entities perform governmental functions, antitrust law may require that the state establish active supervision over their activities. Where state regulation by a private party is involved, and where there is a "gauzy cloak of state involvement over what is essentially a private" anticompetitive activity,[22] the state, in order to obtain antitrust immunity, "must supervise actively" the activity in question.[23] Whether any "anticompetitive" board activities are "essentially" those of private parties depends upon how the regulatory board functions, and perhaps upon the role played by its private members.

Competition Issues Raised by the Activities of Professional Associations and Certifiers of Professional Competence

Associations of professionals engage in a wide variety of activities, including sharing of scientific information, certifying practices and procedures, enunciating standards of practice, verifying the competence of individual practitioners, and propounding codes or norms of conduct. The principal competitive risks associated with private professional associations are that the collective agreements among their members may restrain trade or enable them to monopolize some market for professional services. As discussed below, many such agreements have been the subject of antitrust scrutiny and have spawned a substantial body of law clarifying the boundaries between impermissible cartelization schemes and appropriate trade association activity. A second and more ambiguous area of antitrust concern is the provision by professionals of accrediting or standard-setting services to the market. These activities have potential procompetitive and anticompetitive effects. By improving consumer information, they ameliorate one of the most significant market imperfections and enable buyers and their agents to make more informed judgments. On the other hand, they have the potential to cede de facto control over entry and the nature of clinical practice to private associations, and perhaps to place certain professionals in the position of establishing an "ideological monopoly."[24]

Professional Associations Engaging in Cartelization

Professional groups, including state and national medical associations, trade associations, ad hoc affiliations of doctors, and others, have often adopted rules, norms, edicts, and guidelines that reduce competition among their members. For the most part, these restraints have been treated much like any other horizontal cartel activity under the antitrust laws. These trade restraints have been challenged under a variety of antitrust rubrics: for example, price fixing, market divisions, and boycotts, undertakings that have generally enabled professionals to raise price and reduce output. Courts, economists, and legal commentators regard restraints of this sort as particularly pernicious because demand for healthcare is generally inelastic.[25] Moreover, because of barriers to entry into the professions and economic conditions that limit the ability of consumers to discern quality and select providers, consumers of medical service are generally more vulnerable to victimization by professional cartels.

The first important series of cases in this area involved challenges to "ethical" restrictions imposed by professional associations upon price competition and the contracting practices of their members.[26] Other professional norms (frequently justified by defendants as motivated by quality of care concerns) have been successfully challenged by the government, for example, rules prohibiting physicians from accepting "inadequate" compensation or from "underbidding" other physicians;[27] collective negotiations or threats of boycott by providers against payors or hospitals;[28] and threats by medical staffs of hospitals designed to coerce hospital administrators to abandon plans to open HMOs or recruit new physicians on financial terms objectionable to the staff.[29] In some of these instances, accreditation was a means for effectuating the conspiratorial purpose. For example, in the landmark case *American Medical Association v. United States*,[30] the illegal agreement of the AMA and the Medical Society of the District of Columbia to boycott a group health plan featured threats to hospitals participating in the plan that they would lose AMA approval of their postgraduate physician training programs and threats to participating physicians of loss of AMA and medical society membership.

A second category of cases involves professional association agreements limiting advertising or solicitation of business by members. Unlike the price restraints previously discussed, these restrictions carry at least colorable claims of improving market performance, and their anticompetitive effects are not always facially apparent. However, such restrictions have been routinely struck down as restraints of trade and unfair methods of competition under the antitrust laws, as well as violative of the First

Amendment of the Constitution in certain circumstances.[31] The FTC has enjoined a number of private medical associations from adopting or enforcing ethical codes barring advertising or solicitation.[32] In the leading antitrust case in this area, the FTC challenged the AMA's restrictions on dissemination of price information and ban on advertisements of individual physician's services and alternative forms of care. The FTC concluded that suppression of truthful advertising by doctors was an illegal restraint of trade; however, it approved narrowly tailored ethical restrictions that prohibit advertisements that are false and deceptive.[33] Not only has the government successfully challenged flat bans on advertisements, but it has also found that ethical prohibitions against advertisements mentioning price or discounts, giving information about the practitioner's qualifications, or containing matter deemed undignified or unprofessional violate antitrust laws.[34]

Professional Society Membership and Practice Restrictions

A large part of the raison d'etre of professional societies is the exchange of scientific information and opinion both among members and with buyers and others who lack expertise. In addition, professional society membership often carries with it prestige and may signal that members supply services of high quality or have superior training or expertise. Finally, professional norms and practice parameters may serve the market-improving function of offsetting information deficiencies in the provider-patient relationship.

These potential salutary effects on competitive conditions find doctrinal recognition in antitrust law's rule of reason, which mandates that factfinders assess and balance the procompetitive and anticompetitive effects of horizontal agreements. Weighing on the other side of the ledger are potential cartelizing practices that grow out of standardized professional conduct and exclusionary behavior. For example, membership in a professional society may imply conformance with certain restrictions on the way members compete, and hence raise issues of anticompetitive exclusion or standardization. Profession-imposed standards may ossify practice and reduce innovation. In economic terms, such standards may enable powerful interests to "raise rivals' costs" by denying the acceptance of certain providers by mainstream institutions or forcing them to undertake costly measures to circumvent barriers.

A handful of cases have challenged exclusion from membership in professional societies as a boycott cognizable under the Sherman Act. Courts have rejected these claims where there is no evidence that the exclusion carried with it collateral agreements to standardize medical practice or otherwise limit members' competitive behavior. As one court aptly put it, "it is axiomatic that trade standards must exclude some things as substandard and it is unsurprising that standard-setting bodies sometimes err. A single such error does not amount to a conspiracy."[35] As a general matter, courts have been unwilling to impute anticompetitive effects to the mere denial of membership to a single practitioner in an organization, even where doubts exist as to the professional grounds for the exclusion.[36]

Courts and the FTC have overturned arrangements where professional society membership has carried with it ancillary agreements regarding practice methods that lack any procompetitive justification. For example, trade association rules restricting operation of franchises and branch offices by optometrists, prohibitions against selling products relating to medical services, and prohibitions against affiliations with other providers have been struck down.[37] Nevertheless, where practice restrictions promulgated by a professional society have had plausible justifications based on quality of care, courts have sometimes been willing to take a closer look, though, sometimes nevertheless concluding that the conduct restrained trade. A good example is *Wilk v. American Medical Association*, in which the court grappled with the AMA's prohibitions on all forms of cooperation by medical physicians with chiropractors. The court closely examined the procompetitive justifications, as distinguished from quality of care and "public service" justifications, and found them wanting. In particular, it relied upon evidence that physicians had a specific intent to destroy chiropractors and that there were no procompetitive benefits attributable to the alleged conduct.[38]

Limited quantity-oriented restrictions such as practice guidelines have for the most part escaped sanction, especially where plausible market-improving benefits can be demonstrated or where the society did no more than dispense a collective opinion. For example, a rule promulgated by a society of surgeons mandating that postoperative care be performed only by surgeons was found not violative of the Sherman Act.[39] Courts have readily accepted procompetitive justifications for such conduct. In a case concerning profession-promulgated practice parameters, the actions of a medical specialty society governing the terms and circumstances in which "experimental" procedures should be performed was upheld against the claims that the action constituted concerted activity standardizing a service and limiting interprofessional competition.[40] The case law suggests that the boundary will be drawn to protect "practice guidelines" that enhance information in the market, and that only collective action compelling conformance with society edicts will transgress the antitrust standard.[41]

Certifying, Credentialing, and Peer-Review Activities

By far, the largest number of antitrust cases involving healthcare providers have involved conflicts that, in one way or another, concern professional credentials. These disputes highlight the tension between legitimate professional concerns and the need to prohibit conduct inhospitable to competition. Challenges to denials or curtailment of staff privileges at hospitals have long been a staple of antitrust litigation. In most cases, these disputes have arisen in the context of peer review actions by physician staff members concerning the qualifications, competence, or performance of other providers and their suitability for practice in a hospital. In addition, a number of cases have involved challenges to exclusive contracts with staff-based physicians, such as radiologists, pathologists, and anesthesiologists. In both types of cases, the claim is usually that members of the medical staff either conspired among themselves or conspired with the hospital to exclude a provider or group of providers from membership. In antitrust terms, the activity is generally characterized as a group boycott or, in the case of exclusive contracting, an exclusive dealing or tying arrangement.

Despite the enormous number of staff privilege disputes that have been litigated, only a handful of plaintiffs have succeeded.[42] Courts have held that hospitals have no obligation to admit all licensed practitioners who apply for privileges and have recognized that legitimate, procompetitive impulses usually underlay adverse decisions.[43] As to the question of whether a denial of staff privileges actually restrains trade within the meaning of Section One of the Sherman Act, courts have generally been unwilling to find that such actions violate the antitrust laws absent evidence of an actual anticompetitive effect. Thus, where the hospital denying privileges lacks market power, the cases typically conclude that the plaintiff had other alternatives in the market, or rely on other evidence proving the absence of anticompetitive effect or purpose. In these circumstances, the exclusion has generally been deemed to be "reasonable."[44] Although less frequently litigated, similar challenges to exclusions from provider-controlled payment systems have also been unsuccessful.[45]

However, where the collective refusal to grant privileges constituted either part of a coercive effort against a class of providers (e.g., osteopaths, psychologists, or nurse-midwives) or an attempt to force others to deny staff privileges in order to accomplish an anticompetitive objective, courts have been less reluctant to label the agreement "unreasonable."[46] The case law and commentary support closer scrutiny of "class-based" exclusions for several reasons.[47] First, traditional justifications for privilege denials—that is, those premised on an individual practitioner's competence or record, or the heightened risk of malpractice exposure for the hospital—would not justify excluding an entire group absent evidence tainting the competence of the class of practitioners. Indeed, widespread adoption of policies denying staff privileges to nonphysicians may in some instances thwart competition-enhancing objectives of state licensure laws. Second, commentators have questioned whether physicians are equipped to judge the skill and training of allied practitioners, especially where the privileges in question limit the scope of the latters' practice within the institution. On the other hand, exclusion from access to hospitals may not have a serious effect on certain nonphysician providers where such providers do not need privileges to compete in the market. Moreover, while class-based exclusions may be regarded as suspect, they may be justified by other factors such as a hospital's desire to position itself as a prestigious facility committed to research.

In contrast to the staff privileges cases, the certification activities of private specialty boards and other accrediting groups have produced relatively little antitrust litigation. Certification activities may in theory pose competitive issues when the certifying entity is controlled by competitors. In such circumstances, the controlling practitioners may be accused of attempting to limit the supply of competitors or maintain an "ideological monopoly" by restricting entry by those who would practice the profession using unorthodox (and perhaps less costly) methods of treatment or diagnosis. However, such cases pose extraordinarily difficult problems for antitrust tribunals because of the uncertain nature of the purported "restraint of trade" involved and the ambiguous dimensions of the "market" that may be affected.

It is important to distinguish between those actions of certifiers that have an effect on the marketplace, as many undoubtedly do, and those that unreasonably restrain trade within the meaning of the antitrust laws. As a general matter, antitrust law prohibits "self-regulation" in the sense that the term implies the exercise of direct and coercive regulation over its members and others. In contrast, certification by itself entails only the promulgation of standards and an attestation of compliance with them, not an agreement to sanction noncompliers.[48] An illustrative case is

Poindexter v. American Board of Surgery,[49] in which the court considered the antitrust claims of a surgeon regarding a board's refusal to certify him in vascular surgery on the ground that he had not completed an accredited vascular surgery fellowship. The court found that plaintiff had not established a restraint of trade because he had failed to rebut the board's showing that its standard setting had served legitimate and beneficial ends that tended to improve, not hinder, competition. Moreover, the board had not itself interfered with plaintiff's ability to practice; instead "users" of the information (hospitals, patients, and insurers) had voluntarily relied on the certification activities of the board. As a general matter, then, certification may be seen as a kind of seal of approval that others may be free to follow or ignore; thus, certifiers have not agreed to restrain trade within the meaning of the Sherman Act, but have merely issued a collective opinion upon which others may act.[50] While accreditors have occasionally run afoul of antitrust law, it has usually been because of collateral agreements they have undertaken (such as to boycott or sanction those not meeting the accreditors' standards), rather than the mere adoption of standards and certification of compliance.

A second level of analysis may be necessary to ensure that the certifiers have not corrupted the competitive market by putting forth misleading, deceptive, or fraudulent information.[51] In principle, such activities should be within the ambit of antitrust consideration, but only if the certifiers were able to turn information imperfections in the market to their advantage through a collective agreement to put out distortive information. This inquiry may pose difficult problems in litigation: Courts would be required to evaluate the merits of the information supplied, a task that the litigation process is ill suited to perform.

Finally, it has been suggested that the problem should be framed in terms of examining the effects of competitor-sponsored credentialing and certification on the "market for information."[52] Rather than focus on the actions of accrediting organizations, this approach emphasizes that joint ventures combining the most likely competitors in the production of information through accreditation might be the subject of challenge as an illegal monopoly or restraint of trade. In effect, the claim would be that the sponsors of the accrediting organization should in some cases be "broken up" into smaller aggregations so that multiple accreditors would compete to provide these services. Organizations such as the JCAHO (a joint venture of the AMA, the American Hospital Association (AHA), two prominent medical associations, and others); the Advisory Board for Medical Specialties (ABMS) (twenty-four medical specialty boards and six national organizations); and the Liaison Committee on Medical Education (the AMA and the Association of Medical Colleges) are suggested as potential targets.[53]

Third Parties Adopting the Standards of Private Boards and Associations

When third parties (e.g., payors, hospitals, employers, or networks) use standards adopted by accreditors, there is relatively little risk of challenge under the antitrust laws. As an initial matter, the mere adoption of standards promulgated by a professional organization does not amount to a "combination or conspiracy" under Section One of the Sherman Act. For example, in *Virginia Academy of Clinical Psychologists v. Blue Shield of Virginia*,[54] a physicians' specialty society had recommended to two payment plans that they refuse to reimburse covered members directly for the services of psychologists. The court found that the society's urging the position did not amount to an agreement and underscored the society's freedom to advocate its position as long as it exerted no coercion on others to follow the recommendation.[55]

Moreover, the action of the specialty society may not constitute a restraint of trade where, in fact, nothing more was done than to provide information to a third party. For example, in *Schachar v. American Academy of Ophthalmology*,[56] the court upheld the actions of the Academy in recommending that a procedure be treated as "experimental" and urging that it be approached "with caution" until additional research was completed. While the Academy's actions undoubtedly had an important effect on the ability of competing ophthalmologists to perform the procedure since most insurers deny reimbursement for experimental procedures, the collective provision of an opinion did not constitute a "restraint" of trade. As Judge Easterbrook framed the test, "when a trade association provides information but does not constrain others to follow its recommendations, it does not violate the antitrust laws."[57]

Finally, reliance by third parties on the standards set by a specialty board may well supply evidence of the procompetitive effects of a collective action analyzed under the rule of reason. For example, in *Flegel v. Christian Hospital Northeast-Northwest*,[58] a hospital made board certification by an ABMS-certified board (or eligibility for same) a prerequisite for obtaining staff privileges. The court upheld the arrangement, finding that the agreement to condition privileges did not constitute a per se violation and suggested that the requirements might even help satisfy the defendants' burden under the rule of reason, since it underscored the hospitals' procompetitive rationale of enhancing its reputation and improving quality of service.[59]

Appraising Antitrust's Role

The foregoing section indicates that antitrust law takes some rather intricate turns when dealing with professional self-regulation and certification. The law in this area perhaps can be best understood as an attempt to accommodate numerous conflicting policies and legal doctrines that complicate applying traditional microeconomic principles to matters that concern quality of care and professionalism.

Regulation by governmental entities, including both licensure and explicit governmental deference to private bodies, is well insulated from antitrust scrutiny. Although in extreme cases, such as fraudulent misrepresentation of facts to governmental agencies, or "sham" petitioning, private parties may incur antitrust liability, most quality-related interventions by government are immune. This is true even though such actions may serve private interests, impair competition, or otherwise harm consumer interests. The limitation on antitrust's scope is based on well-founded concerns about the judiciary's capacity (and legitimacy) to review policy choices inherent in certification and standard setting. In addition, considerations of federalism and First Amendment rights to petition the government limit the intrusion of antitrust into governmental activities. Nevertheless, some may question whether judicial deference has gone too far. Discussing the problem in the context of accreditation of health care institutions, Professor Havighurst has written:

> If antitrust law can neither prevent nor counteract the effects of a failure by the political-economic system to resolve an issue democratically either by legislative action or by consumer choice in the marketplace, then private interests will have many opportunities to use private accrediting to shape their legal, regulatory, and economic environments and to control the options available to consumers. To be sure, political institutions ultimately oversee the actions of private accreditors. But political pressures and the inherent limitations of collective action and public choice systematically incline such institutions toward serving special and majoritarian interests rather than the interests of individual consumers.[60]

Where governmental involvement is lacking, the story is quite different. Professional associations come under close antitrust scrutiny when they engage in collective decision making for their members with the purpose or effect of reducing competition. The law affords virtually no leniency in recognition of worthy purposes (such as advancing quality of care), not-for-profit status, or knowledge-advancing objectives of a learned profession. Like the law's deference to governmental actions, the stringency of this approach is also rooted in reservations about judicial capacity to perform a complex balancing of competing social objectives. These concerns are well founded. Were courts required to take into account such concerns, they would face a series of unanswerable questions with no principles to guide them. What kind of professional concerns qualify for special treatment? How much quality protection or professional leeway is required to trump substantial competitive restraints? Given the elastic nature of the concepts involved (quality of care and professionalism), can these benefits be estimated, much less weighed, against consumer harms flowing from the lessened competition?

At the same time, one must question whether the law has unnecessarily blinded itself to the complexities of healthcare market transactions. There is, in fact, ample support in antitrust doctrine for courts to take into account market imperfections when weighing the effects of collective action by professionals. Thus, information-improving collaboration that might otherwise be regarded as a restraint of trade might be excused if, on balance, the improvement in market functioning outweighs all potential harms.[61] This inquiry would maintain the law's proper focus on competitive conditions, but would broaden its scope to take into account serious information deficiencies that affect real-world transactions. To give one example, profession-sponsored restrictions on solicitation may be justified in certain circumstances, such as when they reduce deceptive or fraudulent information or information directed at a vulnerable population. In these circumstances, a court might take into account the extent of information deficits in the market and the fact that restricting such advertising or solicitation improves the market's functioning by preventing tainted or abusive practices from poisoning the entire market.[62]

As noted, competitor-controlled standard setting and certification occupy a gray area in antitrust jurisprudence. Although risks are undoubtedly present, as dominant professional groups might put forward inaccurate, misleading, or biased information that disfavors certain practitioners, serious practical and theoretical problems weigh against antitrust activism in this area. A principal difficulty is whether courts are competent to conduct an inquiry at the heart of which are questions of scientific method, disputed and complex epidemiological data, and divergent professional opinion. More fundamentally, where the standard or certification has been freely accepted by third parties, an open question exists as to whether the professional sponsors should be held liable because it is, after all, the adoption of the standard by payors, hospitals, and others that inflicts the injury on disfavored providers. A pure Chicago-school microeconomic approach says "no." In *Schachar*, Judge

Easterbrook expressed this viewpoint, observing that the Academy's guidelines on radial keratotomy "affected only the demand side of the market, and then only by appealing to consumers' (and third party payers') better judgment. If such statements should be false or misleading or incomplete or just plain mistaken, the remedy is not antitrust litigation but more speech—the marketplace of ideas."[63] This approach may be faulted for unnecessarily cabining antitrust's scope. It assumes that economic coercion operates only when conspirators take steps to impose sanctions or prevent third parties from acting in a certain way. Because, as the Supreme Court put it, "agreement on a product standard is, after all, implicitly an agreement not to manufacture, distribute, or purchase certain types of products,"[64] such activities may well carry the requisite collaborative elements and potential competitive harm to invoke antitrust scrutiny in certain cases.[65]

The development of multiple accreditors would obviate many of the competitive concerns discussed above. Indeed, although once thought impractical, multiple accreditation is developing for home health agencies, managed care organizations, and specialty board certification.[66] It is far from clear, however, whether a multiplicity of accreditation sources is good public policy or whether antitrust law is an appropriate vehicle for moving the industry in that direction. As to the advisability of multiple accreditors, Timothy S. Jost has questioned whether accreditors might compete to have the most relaxed standards or be the least intrusive and whether accreditors might develop dependent relationships with accredited institutions.[67] Whether a "race to the bottom" will occur seems likely to depend on the vigilance of third party payors and other consumers of accreditation services. The flurry of quality monitoring by these entities and the rapid development of databases on provider behavior and credentials suggests that independent verification of profession-sponsored accreditors may become feasible. The proposal that antitrust litigation should be used in some cases to promote diverse sources of accreditation,[68] although conceptually sound, is probably impractical, as evidenced by the unwillingness of federal enforcement authorities to undertake such litigation. For example, proving that an accreditor had market power in the "market for accrediting information" would entail enormous difficulties of proof, as courts would require careful delineation of the dimensions of that market, identification of actual and potential competitors, and measurement of the dominant entity's power, or marketshare.[69] No court has recognized such markets, and commentators have questioned proposals to define similar markets that are not linked directly to services or products.

Conclusion

Antitrust has played a modest role in supervising private certification and credentialing in healthcare. On the whole, the law has struck a reasonable balance by prohibiting coercion by provider-controlled bodies while encouraging professionals' freedom to express openly their expert opinions and to advance science-based standards and protocols. Although market forces have recently spurred greater attention from third party payors to these issues, it would be premature to assume that private cartelization schemes will disappear without effective legal remedies.

Notes

1. T. S. Jost. 1995. "Oversight of the Quality of Medical Care: Regulation, Management or the Market?" *Arizona Law Review* 37 (3): 825.

2. R. C. Derbyshire. 1969. *Medical Licensure and Discipline in the United States.* Westport, CT: Greenwood Press.

3. Jost, "Oversight of the Quality of Medical Care," 834 (noting that physicians remained free of hierarchical controls and dominated state medical boards and federal peer review organizations, which "applied standards prescribed by physicians").

4. I. Horowitz. 1980. "The Economic Foundations of Self-Regulation in the Professions." In *Regulating the Professions*, edited by R. D. Blair and S. Rubin, 6–8. Lexington, MA: Lexington Books.

5. Jost, "Oversight of the Quality of Medical Care," 827–35; P. Starr. 1982. *The Social Transformation of American Medicine*. New York: Basic Books, Inc.

6. The Advisory Board of Medical Specialties is a comprehensive private system to train and credential specialists in the absence of government regulation. The board recognizes twenty-four specialty boards that assess a physician's skills through evaluation and examination. Successful candidates are considered "board-certified" specialists, although the process is voluntary and not legally required to practice medicine in any state; see J. J. Smith. 1993. "The Specialty Boards and Antitrust: A Legal Perspective." *Journal of Contemporary Health Law and Policy* 10 (Spring): 195.

7. The Liaison Committee on Medical Education accredits medical schools and includes representatives of the AMA, the Association of American Medical Colleges, the Committee for Accreditation of Canadian Medical Schools, the federal government, and medical students.) The Accreditation Council for Graduate Medical Education accredits residency programs and comprises representatives from the AMA, the Association of American Medical Colleges, the ABMS, the AHA, and the Council of Medical Specialty Societies, as well as nonvoting representatives of the public and federal government.

8. The JCAHO is a joint venture of the AMA, the AHA, physician organizations, and others. Its operations have been dominated by physicians, according to commentators. C. C. Havighurst and P. M. Brody. 1994. "Accrediting and the Sherman Act," *Law and Contemporary Problems* 57 (Autumn): 240.

9. Jost, "Oversight of the Quality of Medical Care," 836–37; A. Relman. 1988. "Assessment and Accountability: The Third Revolution in Medical Care." *New England Journal of Medicine* 319 (18): 1220.

10. *United States v. Grinnell Corporation*, 384 U.S. 563 (1966).

11. Private parties injured in their business or property may recover treble damages, costs, and attorneys' fees for antitrust violations. 15 U.S.C. § 15.

12. See *Brown Shoe v. United States*, 370 U.S. 294 (1962).

13. *National Society of Professional Engineers v. United States*, 435 U.S. 679 (1978).

14. A suggestive footnote in *Goldfarb v. Virginia State Bar*, 421 U.S. 773, 778–79 (n. 17) intimated that "it would be unrealistic to view the practice of professions as interchangeable with other business activities" and stated that "the public service aspect, and other features of the professions, may require that a particular practice, which could properly be viewed as a violation of the Sherman Act in another context, be treated differently." Despite this language, however, the Supreme Court has repeatedly refused to allow "professional" concerns, or public service, safety, or quality of care factors to outweigh anticompetitive harms in a series of cases involving medical and other professions. See, e.g., *F.T.C. v. Indiana Fed. of Dentists*, 476 U.S. 447 (1986); *Arizona v. Maricopa County Medical Society*, 457 U.S. 332 (1982). See generally, T. L. Greaney. 1989. "Quality of Care and Market Failure Defenses in Antitrust Health Care Litigation." *Connecticut Law Review* 21 (3): 605–65.

15. *California Retail Liquor Dealers v. Midcal Aluminum, Inc.*, 445 U.S. 97, 105 (1980).

16. *Eastern R.R. Presidents Conference v. Noerr Motor Freight, Inc.*, 365 U.S. 127 (1961).

17. *City of Columbia v. Omni Outdoor Advertising, Inc.*, 494 U.S. 365 (1991); *Potters Medical Center v. City Hospital Association*, 800 F.2d 568 (6th Cir. 1986).

18. *Murphy v. Aetna Life & Casualty*, 1988-2 Trade Cas. (CCH) para. 68,240 (D.Or. 1986).

19. *Konecke v. Medical Service*, 1975 Trade Cas. (CCH) para. 60,459 (D.D.C. 1975) (Medicare peer reviewers functioning as agents for federal government immune). Moreover, Congress clearly has the power to exempt certain conduct or even whole industries from the applicability of federal and state antitrust statutes, although such exemptions are not lightly inferred. See *United States v. American Telephone & Telegraph Co.*, 461 F.Supp. 1314 (D.D.C. 1978); *National Gerimedical Hospital & Gerontology Center v. Blue Cross*, 452 U.S. 378 (1981).

20. See *United States v. Texas State Board of Public Accountancy*, 464 F.Supp. 400 (W.D. Tex. 1978), aff'd with modifications per curiam, 592 F.2d 919 (5th Cir.), cert. denied, 444 U.S. 925 (1979); *FTC v. Monahan*, 832 F.2d 688 (1st Cir. 688) (enforcing FTC subpoena against state board of registration in pharmacy despite claim of state action immunity).

21. See *Sessions Tank Liners, Inc. v. Joor Manufacturing, Inc.*, 17 F.3d 295 (9th Cir.), cert. denied, U.S. (1994). Cf. *Allied Tube & Conduit Corp. v. Indian Head, Inc.*, 486 U.S. 492 (1988).

22. *California Retail Liquor Dealers Association v. Midcal Aluminum, Inc.*, 445 U.S. 97, 106, 100 S.Ct. 937, 943, 63 L.Ed.2d 233 (1980)

23. *Southern Motor Carriers Rate Conference, Inc. v. United States*, 471 U.S. 48, 57, 105 S.Ct. 1721, 1727, 85 L.Ed.2d 36 (1985)

24. C. C. Havighurst and N. M. P. King. 1983. "Private Credentialing of Health Care Personnel: An Antitrust Perspective." *American Journal of Law and Medicine* (Parts One and Two): 131, 189, 263.

25. B. R. Furrow, T. L. Greaney, S. H. Johnson, T. S. Jost, and R. L. Schwartz. 1995. *Health Law* vol. 1. St. Paul, MN: West Publishing, § 10-4; J. E. Lopatka. 1991. "Antitrust and Professional Rules: A Framework for Analysis." *San Diego Law Review* 28 (2): 301.

26. The federal courts and the FTC challenged the AMA's rules condemning physicians associating with HMOs and collective activity denying staff privileges and imposing other sanctions on those members who in any way assisted innovative financing and delivery plans. See, e.g., *American Medical Association v. United States*, 317 U.S. 519 (1943); *Group Health Cooperative of Puget Sound v. King County Medical Society*, 237 P.2d 737 (Wash. 1951).

27. See, e.g, American Medical Association, 94 F.T.C. 701 (1979) (consent order).

28. Michigan State Medical Society, 101 F.T.C. 191 (1983) (striking down attempt by physicians to deal collectively with state, Medicaid, and Blue Shield payment systems through group negotiations and threats of "departicipation").

29. S. A. Hope, M.D., 98 F.T.C. 58 (1981); Medical Staff of Prince Georges County, 110 F.T.C. 476 (1988) (consent order).

30. 317 U.S. 519 (1943).

31. See *Peel v. Attorney Registration and Disciplinary Commission of Illinois*, 496 U.S. 91 (1990). *Virginia State Board of Pharmacy v. Virginia Citizens Consumer Council Inc.*, 425 U.S. 748 (1976).

32. See, e.g., *In re California Dental Association* (Docket No. 9259), March 25, 1996 (slip opinion); Michigan Optometric Association, 106 F.T.C. 342 (1985) (consent order).

33. See generally American Medical Association, 94 F.T.C. 701 (1979) (consent order).

34. See, e.g., Connecticut Chiropractor Association, 56 Fed.Reg. 23586 (1991) (consent order).

35. *Consolidated Metals Products v. American Petroleum Institution*, 846 F.2d 284, 294 (5th Cir. 1988).

36. See *Marrese v. American Academy of Orthopedic Surgeons*, 977 F.2d 585 (7th Cir. 1992).

37. See, e.g., American Academy of Ophthalmologists, 108 F.T.C. 25 (1986); Michigan Optometric Association, 106 F.T.C. 342 (1985); Iowa Chapter of the American Physical Therapy Association, No. C-3242 (1988) (consent order).

38. See *Wilk v. American Medical Association*, 895 F.2d 352 (7th Cir.), cert. denied, 496 U.S. 927 (1990).

39. See *Koefoot v. American College of Surgeons*, 652 F.Supp. 882 (N.D. Ill. 1986).

40. *Schachar v. American Academy of Ophthalmology*, 870 F.2d 397 (7th Cir. 1989).

41. Ibid.

42. See, e.g., *Boczar v. Manatee Hospitals & Health System, Inc.*, 993 F.2d 1514 (11th Cir. 1993); see generally B. Furrow, T. Greaney, S. Johnson, T. Jost, and R. Schwartz. 1994. *Health Care*. St. Paul, MN: West Publishing, ch. 10.

43. See, e.g., *Kaczanowshki v. Medical Center Hospital*, 612 F.Supp. 688 (D.Vt. 1985); see generally B. Furrow et al., *Health Law*, supra note §§ 10-16, 10-24.

44. See, e.g., *Bhan v. NME Hospitals, Inc.*, 929 F.2d 1404 (9th Cir.), cert. denied 112 S.Ct. 617 (1991); *Goss v. Memorial Hospital Systems*, 789 F.2d 353 (5th Cir. 1986).

45. *Hassan v. Independent Practice Associations*, 698 F.Supp. 679 (E.D. Mich. 1988).

46. See, e.g., *American Medical Association v. United States*, 317 U.S. 519; *Oltz v. St. Peter's Community Hospital*, 861 F.2d 1440 (9th Cir. 198); *Weiss v. York Hospital*, 745 F.2d 786 (3d Cir. 1984), cert. denied, 470 U.S. 1060 (1985).

47. See Note. G. Reindl. 1986. "Denying Hospital Privileges to Non-Physicians: Does

Quality of Care Justify a Potential Restraint of Trade?" *Indiana Law Review* 19 (4): 1219; P. Kissam, W. Webber, L. Bigus, and J. Holzgraefe. 1982. "Antitrust and Hospital Privileges: Testing the Conventional Wisdom." *California Law Review* 70 (3): 595; J. F. Blumstein and F. A. Sloan. 1988. "Antitrust and Peer Review." *Law and Contemporary Problems* 51 (Spring): 7.

48. Havighurst and Brody, "Accrediting and the Sherman Act," 212.

49. 911 F.Supp. 1510 (N.D. Ga. 1994).

50. Schachar, 870 F.2d at 399 (no restraint of trade where professional society's standard setting had not "prevented [anyone] from doing what he wished" or imposed sanctions).

51. See Havighurst and Brody, "Accrediting and the Sherman Act," 228 (advocating a rational basis test that would impose limited antitrust review on accrediting decisions, inquiring whether "there are overt signs that the collaborators were not, in fact, primarily interested in informing interested parties of the relative merits of certain goods and services [and intervening if] the parties were . . . trying to deceive . . . customers, to manipulate an unresponsive government program, or to exploit some other market imperfection.")

52. Havighurst and King, "Private Credentialing," C. C. Havighurst. 1988. "Applying Antitrust Law to Collaboration in the Production of Information: The Case of Medical Technology Assessment." *Law & Contemporary Problems* 51 (Winter): 341.

53. Havighurst and Brody, "Accrediting and the Sherman Act," 228.

54. 624 F.2d 476 (4th Cir. 1980), cert. denied, 450 U.S. 916 (1981).

55. Ibid.

56. 879 F.2d 397 (7th Cir. 1989).

57. Ibid., at 399.

58. 804 F.Supp. 1165 (E.D. Mo. 1992), aff'd 4 F. 3d 682 (8th Cir. 1993).

59. Ibid.

60. Havighurst and Brody, "Accrediting and the Sherman Act," 211.

61. See T. L. Greaney. 1989. "Quality of Care." *Connecticut Law Review* 21 (3): 605–65.

62. Ackerlof. 1970. "The Market for Lemons: Quality, Uncertainty and the Market Mechanism." *Quarterly Journal of Economics* 24: 488.

63. Schachar, 879 F.2d, at 400.

64. *Allied Tube & Conduit Corp. v. Indian Head, Inc.*, 486 U.S. 492, 500 (1988). See Havighurst and Brody, "Accrediting and the Sherman Act," 214–16.

65. See Furrow et al. *Health Law*, § 10-14b.

66. T. S. Jost. 1994. "Medicare and the Joint Commission on Accreditation of Healthcare Organizations: A Healthy Relationship?" *Law and Contemporary Problems* 57 (Autumn): 15.

67. T. S. Jost, "Medicare and the Joint Commission," 43–45. For a critical account of many nontraditional boards and the American Federation of Medical Accreditation, an organization that accredits them, see K. Terry. 1995. "Visit Las Vegas! Get Your Boards while You're There." *Medical Economics* 72 (3): 26.

68. Havighurst and Brody, "Accrediting and the Sherman Act"; Havighurst and King, "Private Credentialing of Health Care Personnel: An Antitrust Perspective."

69. For a discussion of how these problems might be resolved, see Havighurst and Brody, "Accrediting and the Sherman Act," 236–38.

THE EBB AND FLOW OF FEDERAL INITIATIVES TO REGULATE HEALTHCARE PROFESSIONALS

Mark R. Yessian and Joyce M. Greenleaf*

Backdrop

Bias Toward Inaction

On most domestic matters, the federal government functions with a strongly rooted bias toward inaction. This bias reflects traditional American values of individualism and limited government. It is sustained by the warnings of founding fathers such as Thomas Jefferson, who in a 1787 letter to James Madison acknowledged, "I am not a friend to a very energetic government. . . . It is always oppressive."[1] More significantly, the U.S. Constitution reinforces this bias by separating the powers of the federal government among executive, legislative, and judicial branches, and by establishing a federal system of governance, with state governments possessing all those powers not specifically provided to the national government.

On matters pertaining to the federal regulation of health professionals, the bias toward inaction has been reinforced further by the long-standing norms of professionalism. Through these norms, professionals, particularly physicians, have enjoyed far-reaching discretion. Society, in effect, has been willing to defer to their expertise and judgment, with the

---

*The views expressed in this chapter are those of the authors and do not necessarily represent those of the Office of Inspector General or the U.S. Department of Health and Human Services.

tacit understanding that they will give primacy to an ethic of service, as is most clearly reflected by the Hippocratic oath.[2] To the extent professionals have been regulated in the United States, for instance through licensure laws, that regulation historically has been at the state level.

Basis for Federal Initiatives to Regulate Health Professionals

In this milieu, how, then, can the fact that from time to time the federal government has regulated and to some degree diminished the discretion of professionals be explained? Many forces have contributed, but two have been prominent: cost containment and consumer protection. When the federal government pays for some or all of costs of professional care, the need to exert some control over those costs can become compelling, especially during periods when costs escalate rapidly. Whether or not the federal government is the payor, the need to protect consumers from harm can also become compelling, particularly when evidence accumulates that protection is not adequately afforded by state regulation or by professional self-regulation.[3]

At those times when the federal government moves to regulate healthcare professionals, either or both of the two above noted forces are almost certainly involved in providing the motivating rationale. Policymakers become sufficiently alarmed about program costs, consumer risks, or both to summon the resolve to break through the traditional restraints exerted by American beliefs and by professionalism.

Introduction of Medicare and Medicaid

In 1965, in order to provide many Americans with better access to healthcare, Congress enacted the Medicare and Medicaid programs.[4] Both programs were adopted despite strong objections by medical professionals and by those arguing for state-based approaches to improve access. With much accumulated evidence regarding the unmet health needs of the elderly, disabled, and poor, the perceived need for federal action was strong enough to override the widely expressed objections.[5]

With respect to Medicare, popular support to assist the elderly was strong enough to warrant a federal, single-payor program, albeit one that incorporated many compromises to make it palatable enough to gain sufficient backing among medical professionals, states, and others uneasy about this significant extension of federal authority. Among the myriad compromises that limited the role of the federal government were the payment for physician services on the basis of "reasonable and necessary" charges; the review and processing of Medicare claims for services by private insurance companies; the reliance on states to determine if physicians met the minimum necessary qualifications to practice; and the prohibition of any federal intrusion into the "routine practice of medicine."

With respect to Medicaid, the support for federal action to assist the poor, even in the midst of President Johnson's "War on Poverty" was too fragile to permit a comparable national initiative, even with compromises such as those noted above. Here, the result was a federal-state program that established certain minimum federal requirements, but gave the states significant latitude to determine eligibility, covered services, payments to providers, and other matters.

As Medicare and Medicaid grew over the years, the federal government became increasingly concerned about cost and quality issues and enacted many laws and regulations that in some way regulated the practice of healthcare professionals. Some addressed the policies and conditions of facilities in which health professionals practiced, such as federal actions regulating hospitals, nursing homes, dialysis centers, dental offices, and clinical laboratories. Some established review mechanisms intended to halt the proliferation of expensive medical facilities and technologies. Some put in place external review mechanisms to determine the necessity and adequacy of services being provided by physicians and other caregivers. Some even focused on financial conflicts of interest, as in the case of laws concerning kickbacks and self-referrals of patients.[6]

Each of these laws was justified on the basis of perceived needs to protect taxpayers, patients, or both. Each, in effect, reflected some dissatisfaction with protections afforded by the professional norms of practice, professional associations, and state governments. Each somehow was enacted and enforced despite deep-seated barriers to federal regulation of professionals.

This Chapter

This chapter focuses on three significant federal initiatives that regulate healthcare professionals: one that focuses on Medicare, one that focuses on Medicaid, and one that reaches across both programs and the healthcare sector more broadly. Each was passed by Congress to help contain costs, protect the public, or both. Each emerged from a sense of taxpayer or consumer vulnerabilities significant enough to galvanize national action. The three federal initiatives are: (1) the Medicare Peer Review Program; (2) the Medicaid drug utilization review requirements; and (3) the National Practitioner Data Bank. In each case, the chapter will examine the rationale giving rise to the legislation, review the evolution of the initiative since its passage by Congress, and assess the state of the initiative at a time when federal regulation of any kind remains highly suspect. Throughout, the intent will be to help elucidate the factors that affect the ebb and flow of federal initiatives to regulate healthcare professionals.

With the same intent, the chapter will also examine briefly three failed federal initiatives to regulate healthcare professionals. Each was incorporated into proposed legislation. Each sought to protect consumers from harm, and one also aimed, indirectly, to contain costs as well. Yet, each failed to attract sufficient support to become enacted. The three are: (1) the 1990 proposal to mandate physician credentialing; (2) the 1994 proposal to provide federal grants for state medical boards; and (3) the 1994 proposal to override state professional licensure laws under particular circumstances.

Enacted Federal Initiatives

The Medicare Peer Review Organization Program

Rationale

By the early 1970s, Medicare costs were accelerating. Expenditures had nearly tripled from about $3.3 billion in 1967 to $9.5 billion in 1973. In response, Congress created the Professional Standards Review Organization (PSRO) program to determine whether services paid for by Medicare were medically necessary, met professional standards, and were provided in appropriate settings. In deference to the medical community, Congress mandated that PSROs be local, physician-sponsored organizations. Before long, 203 PSROs were operating across the country.

By the early 1980s, the PSRO program was on shaky ground. Physician irritation with PSROs as an external review entity was mounting. Medicare expenditures continued to rise—to $50 billion by 1982. The General Accounting Office (GAO) and Congressional Budget Office each came out with reports critical of the PSRO program and its cost effectiveness.[7] The AMA called for its repeal. And it fell under the scrutiny of the newly elected Reagan Administration that sought to sweep away excessive regulation.

But, unlike other federal regulatory programs of that era, such as health planning, the PSRO program managed to survive. By reincarnating it in 1982 into a leaner, meaner, and more accountable program, Senator David Durenberger essentially saved it.[8] No longer called the PSRO program, it was now the Utilization and Quality Peer Review Organization (PRO) program.[9]

The PRO program that emerged was less deferential to the medical profession than its predecessor. Congress continued to require that local physicians conduct the medical reviews, but it replaced the local PSROs with statewide PROs. In testimony before Congress, the AMA expressed its displeasure, noting that the PRO program "would continue many of the objectionable features of the existing PSRO program" and would "present a potential improper intrusion into the physician's practice."[10]

Evolution

Seven months after the program was enacted, Congress adopted a bold new approach to paying for inpatient hospital care for Medicare beneficiaries. In place of the traditional retrospective payment system, it established a prospective payment system (PPS) based on diagnosis related groups (DRGs).[11] It recognized that PPS introduced an incentive for underutilization, with the possibility that beneficiaries would be discharged "quicker and sicker," and it looked to the PROs to serve as safety valves. It called for the PROs, through contracts with hospitals, to provide an independent assessment of the completeness, adequacy, and quality of care provided under PPS.

Thus the PRO program shifted course from one focused on cost control to one aimed at consumer protection. Additional legislative mandates reinforced this shift. In 1985, Congress authorized the PROs to deny payment for care they determined to be of a substandard quality.[12] In 1986, Congress mandated that "a reasonable proportion" of PROs' review activities be involved with quality; that PROs review written, quality-related beneficiary complaints; and that PRO boards include at least one consumer representative.[13] The AMA objected to the inclusion of a consumer on the PRO boards.[14]

Like the PSRO program it replaced, the PRO program came under external scrutiny. In 1988 and 1989, the Office of Inspector General (OIG) of the Department of Health and Human Services (HHS) issued reports charging that the PROs were largely unsuccessful in identifying poor quality care and in holding physicians accountable for such care once identified.[15]

During this period, the relationship between the PROs and the medical community became more adversarial than ever. As called for in their contracts with the Health Care Financing Administration (HCFA), PROs were tracking and scoring by severity individual quality-of-care problems identified during medical record reviews.[16] Based on these efforts, they would take follow-up actions intended to educate or punish individual physicians and hospitals.

This aspect of the PROs' performance—the focus on identifying and responding to individuals responsible for questionable care—left virtually no one happy. The medical community complained that the focus was "highly offensive" as it was overly punitive and added needless hassle to the practice of medicine.[17] At the same time, the OIG and others looking to PROs to protect patients from harm found fault with the lenient follow-up actions the PROs took when they identified quality-of-care problems. The majority of actions consisted simply of notification, educational letters, or telephone calls.[18] The PROs rarely shared case information with state medical licensure boards.[19] And they almost never took the most severe action available to them, referral to the OIG for sanction.[20]

Meanwhile, the concept of quality assurance in healthcare was undergoing profound change. Emphasis was shifting from the focus on individual providers and quality-of-care problems to systems of care, borrowing from the TQM school of thought.[21] This school of thought holds that it is far more important to focus on improving the mainstream of care than on identifying and responding to poor performers at the margin.

The PROs' focus was clearly out of sync with this new approach to quality. And in 1990, the Institute of Medicine (IOM) pointed this out in an influential assessment of Medicare quality assurance efforts.[22] It questioned the effect of the PROs and urged a major redirection of their efforts along the lines of a CQI model.

In response to the IOM and the extensive criticism from the medical community, HCFA completely changed the focus of the PRO program in 1993.[23] Noting that the PROs were "seen as largely ineffective," HCFA called for them to "forge new relationships with the medical community" to improve care.[24] Now called the Health Care Quality Improvement Program (HCQIP), the new PRO program stressed collaboration rather than confrontation. Instead of identifying and addressing individual clinical problems through medical record review, PROs would now aim to improve the overall practice of medicine by analyzing patterns of care and outcomes and sharing information with the medical community.[25]

Unlike the many changes to the PRO program throughout the 1980s, this profound change occurred without any new mandate from Congress; Congress held hearings but passed no new legislation.[26] While the medical community welcomed this shift in focus by the PROs, others were somewhat uneasy. For example, the American Association of Retired Persons (AARP), while lauding the shift toward improved care overall, noted that "the Medicare program must continue to protect beneficiaries from poor care."[27] The OIG also expressed concern. Like the AARP, it recognized the promise of the new direction, but in a 1995 report questioned the PROs' ability to identify, let alone respond to, poorly performing physicians and hospitals given their new focus.[28] The GAO reiterated this concern in a later report.[29]

Assessment

In its 25-year history, the PSRO/PRO program has been strongly affected by the ebb and flow of political concerns about the Medicare program. During its first decade or so of operation, it concentrated on cost savings, then evolved in the late 1980s toward a more consumer-protection orientation, and in the mid-1990s, to yet another focus— improving the mainstream of care for Medicare beneficiaries.

From one perspective, the PROs are now in prime position to gain continued federal support and to serve as a major component of Medicare's quality assurance efforts in the years ahead. They are fixed on the lofty and highly desirable goal of improving medical care in the face of market forces that can pose significant threats to the quality of that care. They are measuring and seeking to improve quality in ways that enjoy strong support in professional quality assurance circles.[30] Not least of all, they are functioning in a less regulatory manner and in more harmony with the medical community than at any time in their history.

From another perspective, however, the PROs' position is much more questionable. At a time when Medicare costs and the long-term viability of the Medicare trust fund are increasingly concerns, the PROs are no longer engaged in containing costs.[31] At a time when Medicare beneficiaries are increasingly enrolling in managed care plans, the PROs have little experience with such plans.[32] At a time when widespread reports of harm caused by medical professionals often generate calls for a governmental response, the PROs are no longer focused on protecting from harm.[33]

It is possible that Congress will be impressed enough with the PROs' performance in contributing to better medical care that the program will be able to establish a secure base. But to the extent Congress finds itself compelled to confront cost or consumer protection concerns, it may look to other entities, create new ones, or, indeed, shift the focus of the PROs once again.

Medicaid Drug Utilization Review Requirements

Rationale

Soon after the passage of the Medicare and Medicaid programs, the concept of drug utilization review (DUR) began to draw attention at the national level. The concept stressed improved drug therapy through the monitoring of prescription drug use.[34] The medical and pharmacy professionals associated with these efforts recognized that improved therapy could save money, but were guarded in suggesting that it could reduce overall prescription drug expenditures.

Impressed by the potential of DUR, the then Department of Health, Education, and Welfare, in 1974, issued regulations calling for the monthly review of prescription drug regimens of Medicaid patients in skilled nursing facilities.[35] During this period, many state Medicaid programs and many private payors were beginning their own DUR efforts, typically quite limited in nature.

In October 1990, following an unsuccessful effort to establish a Medicare DUR program, Congress incorporated a set of DUR requirements into the Medicaid program.[36] The program was part of a package of deficit reduction measures, including Medicaid drug rebate provisions.[37] Congress and the states were concerned about rapidly rising Medicaid expenditures for prescription drugs and clearly expected that the DUR requirements would help contain costs.[38] They were buoyed in this expectation by a Congressional Budget Office projection that a comprehensive DUR effort in just 30 state Medicaid programs would save the state and federal governments $1 billion from 1991 to 1995.[39]

In the statute setting forth the DUR requirements, the cost containment expectations are obscured by language that comes across as much more concerned with quality of care. The statute specified that by January 1, 1993, states were to establish DUR programs for covered outpatient drugs "in order to assure that prescriptions (1) are appropriate, (2) are medically necessary, and (3) are not likely to result in adverse medical results."[40] Toward this end, the states were to carry out programs incorporating: (1) prospective drug review that would allow pharmacists to counsel individuals at the point of drug dispensing; (2) retrospective drug use review that would involve a review of pharmacy claims data to identify inappropriate patterns of physician prescribing, pharmacist dispensing, or patient use; and (3) educational outreach that would contribute to improved professional practice. Although the statute offers no specific statement of intent concerning cost savings, it does call for states to submit annual reports that must estimate cost savings achieved and assess the effect of DUR interventions on the quality of care.

Physicians and pharmacists, the two types of healthcare professionals most affected by this regulation, reacted somewhat differently to it. For physicians, it spelled trouble. Retrospective reviews could add hassle to medical practice, particularly if they led to punitive as well as educational interventions by state Medicaid agencies. Prospective review suggested that pharmacists would become increasingly active in questioning physician prescribing practices.[41] For pharmacists, the prospective review, along with a mandated patient counseling provision, afforded new opportunities for added professional stature, even though pharmacists have often voiced the concern that reimbursement is insufficient to cover counseling services.[42]

In an attempt to harness professional leadership behind the DUR program, Congress mandated that states establish DUR boards to apply DUR standards and oversee DUR interventions. The boards were required to include physicians and pharmacists, but there was no explicit requirement for consumer representation.

Evolution

The states have been the central driving force of the Medicaid DUR program. The federal government has required that states submit annual reports on their programs, but overall has exerted minimal oversight.[43] Even within the states, the DUR programs have generally had a low profile. To the extent they have drawn the attention of policymakers, the interest has centered on potential cost savings. In environments where Medicaid expenditures account for as much as 15 to 20 percent of overall state expenditures and where prescription drug expenditures represent about 7 percent of Medicaid expenditures, this orientation is understandable.[44] As a result, cost savings, rather than improved clinical outcomes, have been the main focus of program evaluations.[45] Moreover, the pressure to show such savings has often led to what some reviewers have concluded are exaggerated, insufficiently documented cost savings.[46]

The most visible manifestation of the DUR programs has been the prospective DUR feature. Most of the states have established statewide, online DUR systems that call for pharmacists to submit Medicaid claims electronically at the time of dispensing. The claims are then screened against a set of criteria, established by the state DUR board, that may serve to disallow a claim or call for further explanation. Denied prescriptions through this pro-DUR process have been major sources of state cost savings claims and of physician and pharmacist irritation with DUR.[47]

Although pro-DUR efforts have been gaining importance, retrospective DUR has remained the main feature of most state programs. These programs involve the review of paid drug claims to identify prescriptions that are not in accord with established drug use criteria. When physicians with questionable prescribing practices are identified, the state agency's intervention is almost always rather genteel. It is likely to involve a letter noting how that physician's practice differs from the established criteria and will often include supporting references to professional literature. Typically, the physician is not even required to reply, although his subsequent prescribing may be reviewed for a period of time to see if the questionable practice changes.

Consumers and consumer organizations are almost totally excluded from this process. Medical and pharmacy professionals (including many in medical and pharmacy schools) have played central roles in implementing the programs for the states. But probably most central have been the commercial vendors states have contracted with to help run their programs. The states typically have depended on these vendors to establish the criteria governing pro-DUR and retrospective DUR efforts and to handle much of the program management and operation, including the estimate of cost savings.[48]

Assessment

At the very core of DUR programs, whether carried out under Medicaid or other payment sources, is an ongoing tension between cost-containment and quality-of-care objectives. Typically, payors and healthcare managers discount the tension by stressing that both objectives are important and compatible. But given the enormous pressures that exist to contain rising healthcare costs, the cost-containment objectives can easily dominate and, in so doing, jeopardize the compatibility of the two objectives.[49]

Given that Medicaid accounts for a much higher proportion of state budgets than of the federal budget, state policymakers are much more likely to look to Medicaid DUR as a cost saver than are their federal counterparts. Whether this has had an adverse effect on quality is unclear. In its review of the first set of DUR annual reports submitted to the federal government by the states, the review team assembled by the American Pharmaceutical Association found that "Assessments of the impact on quality of care were limited to anecdotal evidence."[50]

Notwithstanding the uncertain effect on improving drug therapies, the Medicaid DUR requirements do not appear to have infringed much on professional practice. The pro-DUR component probably has contributed to somewhat greater pharmacist overview of physician prescribing practices and to greater state or vendor input into what prescriptions can be filled. But the retro-DUR efforts have invariably been conducted in a CQI mode, with the aim of improving prescribing and dispensing practices generally rather than of identifying and in some way punishing poor performers. In fact, in accord with strongly stated preferences of the AMA, this kind of "get-the-bad-apples" approach is almost totally absent in the state programs. So, too, is any consumer-directed focus, be it to educate consumers on how to become more informed users of prescription drugs or on how to identify and report professionals who may be causing harm. Professionals, in short, can hardly point to Medicaid DUR as an example of excessive federal regulation diminishing their professional prerogatives.[51]

That would not necessarily be true, however, of DUR as it is being practiced by firms in today's healthcare marketplace. And therein rests the most significant point concerning the outlook for Medicaid DUR and for medical and pharmacy professionals caring for Medicaid beneficiaries. Increasingly, state governments have been looking to that marketplace and in particular to private (usually proprietary) HMOs to manage, on a capitated basis, the healthcare of their Medicaid beneficiaries. These organizations have considerable expertise and experience in the efficient use of healthcare resources, such as hospital emergency rooms, diagnostic tests, or prescription drugs. For the latter, they often contract with pharmaceutical benefit management firms that carefully monitor and even in many respects define prescribing and dispensing practices, with the very explicit intent of saving costs.[52]

If, as seems likely, states continue to look to capitated, comprehensive managed care for their Medicaid beneficiaries, the DUR infrastructure built up by state Medicaid agencies and their vendors could become increasingly irrelevant.[53] For example, in California, about one-half of the more than five million Medicaid beneficiaries must enroll in health plans for most of their medical care, including prescription drugs. For those individuals, the health plans assume the responsibility (and risk) for cost-effective drug therapy. The state oversees the plans, but does not review the prescribing or dispensing practices of individual professionals as it did under the fee-for-service Medicaid program to which the 1990 federal DUR requirements were directed. The managed care DUR that replaces public DUR, however, may in the end prove much more intrusive than the public program.

National Practitioner Data Bank

Rationale

In 1984, the GAO drew national attention to the phenomenon of health-care professionals losing their licenses to practice in one state and then continuing to practice in another. The GAO urged Congress to protect Medicare and Medicaid beneficiaries from such professionals by giving the HHS sufficient authority to exclude them from participating in these national programs. It also called for the HHS inspector general to include all healthcare practitioners sanctioned by state licensing boards in a disciplinary action data bank it was developing.[54]

Within Congress, the report generated considerable attention. Both the Senate and the House of Representatives held hearings focusing on the report and introduced legislation responding to the GAO's recommendations.[55] As it turned out, however, the sense of urgency was not sufficient to support what would be a highly controversial move into a regulatory arena regarded as the province of the states.[56]

Yet, in retrospect, a process was started that would support a significant federal intervention before long. Throughout the country, the media had been giving considerable attention to the dangers the public faced because of incompetent physicians and poorly functioning state licensure boards.[57] Federal and state authorities were also responding. The HHS inspector general issued a widely noted report that raised serious questions about the performance of state medical boards.[58] In New York, California, New Jersey, and many other states, similar reports were issued, questioning the consumer protections afforded by existing regulatory mechanisms.[59]

In the middle of this unsettled situation, a federal court imposed a substantial judgment against 11 Oregon physicians whom the court ruled had violated antitrust laws in carrying out their peer review activities in a clinic in Astoria, Oregon.[60] The judgment triggered widespread alarm among those engaged in professional peer review, setting back efforts at professional self-regulation, and thereby added to the rising sense of public vulnerability to medical incompetence.[61]

This threat to peer review added the ingredient that led to congressional action in 1986. In hearings held during the summer, a House subcommittee received widespread support from the medical community for legislation that would provide liability protections for professionals engaged in peer review. The legislation also called for the HHS secretary to establish a repository for collecting and sharing information on sanctioned practitioners. Among medical professionals, there was clearly much less support for this provision, but, paired as it was with the liability protections, it generated little visible opposition.[62]

Yet, as the 99th Congress was drawing to a close that year and was bogged down in deliberations on the federal budget, it was not at all clear that any legislation extending peer review protections and establishing a national repository would pass. Eventually, largely through the legislative craftsmanship of Congressman Ron Wyden, who represented the Oregon district where the Astoria clinic was located, such legislation did pass. It was entitled the Health Care Quality Improvement Act of 1986 and was incorporated as Title IV of the Omnibus Budget Act of that year.[63]

The legislation required malpractice insurers to report to what came to be called the National Practitioner Data Bank information on all medical malpractice payments they make on behalf of physicians and dentists. It also specified that hospitals, state licensure boards, professional societies, and other healthcare entities report information on adverse actions they take against such practitioners. Further, it mandated that hospitals query this Data Bank for each new appointment to the medical staff, and for every existing staff member once every two years. It authorized, but did not require, certain other entities, such as state licensure authorities, to query the Data Bank.[64]

Evolution

From the beginning, the Data Bank was controversial. The major, initial point of contention was over who would run it.[65] The AMA had made clear during the hearing process that it regarded the Data Bank as unnecessary because it duplicated clearinghouses already being operated by the AMA itself and the Federation of State Medical Boards (FSMB). But, it added, if Congress proceeds to enact a Data Bank requirement, then the responsibility for carrying it out should not be vested in HHS itself "as the track record at HHS does not instill confidence that a system established by HHS would operate properly." The FSMB and others shared this point of view.[66] By December 1988, when HHS hired the Unisys Corporation as the contractor for the Data Bank, both AMA and FSMB were becoming increasingly wary of the new clearinghouse.

In September 1990, nearly four years after the authorizing legislation was enacted, the Data Bank began operation. It did so in the face of an August 1990 GAO report noting insufficient internal controls in the Data Bank and questioning whether it was ready to open.[67] Over the next few years, the Data Bank experienced operational problems that led many reviewers to express serious reservations about its viability. In the spring of 1991, *Medical Economics* published an article under the title, "The Malpractice Data Bank is Turning into a Frankenstein."[68] A year later, *Physician Executive* issued an article, written by a former employee of the Data Bank contractor, with the heading, "Data Bank Incomplete and Future Cloudy."[69] Early the following year, the GAO issued yet another report noting continued problems "that undermine achievement of a timely, secure, and cost-effective operation."[70]

But after two to three years of experience, the tide began to turn and the Data Bank began to function in a much more effective and efficient manner.[71] This progress was recognized in 1993 when the National Practitioner Data Bank won a Federal Leadership Award for "Excellence in Technology."[72] Since then the Data Bank has reduced costs, improved timeliness, and become a reliable central source of information.[73]

With this improvement, the alarm calls about Data Bank management have diminished. But among medical professionals, the very idea of the Data Bank has proved a continuing irritant. A past president of the Idaho Academy of Family Physicians almost certainly reflected the view of most of his colleagues when he said the following about the Data Bank: "I'd like it to just disappear. Let's put it somewhere beyond the reach of fiber optics."[74] The AMA has consistently reflected this sentiment, reaffirming it in a resolution of its House of Delegates in 1995.[75] Among dentists, the same sense of concern has been widely expressed. Indeed, the ADA sued the Data Bank over issues involving the reporting of peer review actions taken by its state dental associations.[76]

In a series of reports, the OIG has shown that as the Data Bank has grown, hospital and managed care officials have found it increasingly useful to them. In these reports, the OIG has also shown that information from the Data Bank actually influenced hospital and managed care organization credentialing decisions about two to three percent of the time.[77] What these data suggest about the effectiveness of the National Practitioner Data Bank is open to interpretation. The AMA argues that they reveal a very minimal effect, supporting its contention that the Data Bank should be terminated. Others indicate that identifying two to three percent could involve the identification of hundreds or even thousands of practitioners who in the course of their practice could endanger thousands of patients.[78]

Even more enduring and volatile than the controversy over the usefulness and effect of the Data Bank is that over whether it should be opened to the public. The controversy was stoked in 1994 when then Congressman (now Senator) Wyden, a Democrat, joined with Congressman Scott Klug, a Republican, to introduce legislation toward that end.[79] The legislation failed to pass, but it led consumer organizations to reaffirm the importance of enabling patients, in an increasingly market-driven healthcare system, to obtain more and better information on the physicians they choose to care for them.[80] At the same time, it reinforced the fears of medical professionals about how information in the Data Bank could be misleading and misused.

Assessment

From the perspective of healthcare professionals, the National Practitioner Data Bank is the boldest and most threatening of the three enacted federal initiatives addressed in this chapter. It is a nationally run program, carried out under uniform, precisely defined rules. It stores potentially damaging information concerning the past practices of tens of thousands of practitioners. Managers in hospitals, managed care organizations, and other healthcare settings use this information to try to identify practitioners who might pose dangers to the public (and to their organizations). Not least of all, pressures have been building to enable patients to gain access to some or all of the information.

The PRO and DUR programs are also bound by many federal rules and offer their own challenges to healthcare professionals. Yet, in contrast, they are relatively benign intrusions. They are carried out in a decentralized manner, the PRO program through about 50 organizations focusing for the most part on individual states and the DUR program by the individual state governments. They are operated under the strong, continuing influence of medical or pharmacy professionals. And their current postures toward quality assurance are clearly to elevate the norms of practice through information sharing and collaboration rather than to protect the public from harm through punitive or rehabilitative efforts directed to poor performers.

Ironically, while the National Practitioner Data Bank represents the most heavy-handed use of federal authority, it is the most in tune with the private market forces transforming the healthcare field.[81] As a result, it may well have more staying power than most professionals would like. The Data Bank, after all, provides an efficient, central source of information to organizations employing healthcare practitioners. Indeed, managed care organizations, which are not now required to query the Data Bank, typically do so and, in fact, have come to account for the majority of queries to the Data Bank.[82]

Over time, physicians and other healthcare professionals may become more accustomed to this intrusion. It will likely be much harder for them to accept the notion that information in the Data Bank should be made available to consumers. But, if we are, indeed, moving toward a consumer-driven healthcare system, as *The Economist* and other sources predict, that, too, is something they could have to get used to before long.[83]

Failed Federal Initiatives

Mandating Physician Recredentialing

During the spring of 1990, as final preparations were being made for the National Practitioner Data Bank, Congressman Pete Stark felt that more needed to be done to protect the public from incompetent physicians. He was concerned that neither state licensure authorities nor private peer-review bodies were sufficiently rigorous in "weeding out doctors who lost their skills or failed to keep up with modern medical practice."[84] So, in

April 1990, Stark proposed that physicians must pass a federally qualified recertification exam at seven-year intervals or be licensed in a state with federally approved, time-limited licensure.[85] His proposal was based on similar plans for periodic recertification in New York.[86] He knew that it had little chance of passage but sought to heighten national attention to the matter. Such attention, he quite likely assumed, could prompt some action by state or private bodies, prepare the groundwork for eventual federal action, or both.[87]

Stark held a hearing on the proposal.[88] Most of the witnesses at the hearing represented medical specialty associations that had their own certification programs. Predictably, they expressed little support for the proposal that they felt would grant too much authority to the federal government and undermine their own certification efforts.[89]

As expected, the legislation failed to pass. In spring 1994, as President Clinton's comprehensive health reform proposal was taking shape, Congressman Stark thought the time for the proposal might have arrived, and introduced the proposal once again. The Clinton proposal would have established a much expanded federal role in the healthcare sector. In that context, it seemed that a measure setting forth a federal mandate for physician recredentialing might not seem as bold as it had four years earlier and might well get incorporated in the comprehensive legislation. But the expectations of the spring were dashed in the fall. The Health Security Act introduced by the President went down amidst a barrage of criticism about its cost, complexity, and reach.[90] And the Stark proposal went down with it.

Overriding State Licensure Laws

Another proposal that had become associated with the Health Security Act would have preempted state licensure laws found to be overly restrictive. Introduced as a section of the Health Security Act, it stated the following: "No State may, through licensure or otherwise, restrict the practice of any class of health professionals beyond what is justified by the skills and training of such professionals."[91]

This legislative provision came from the President's health reform planning effort, from which emerged a concern that restrictive scope-of-practice provisions of state licensure laws could be more protective of healthcare professionals than of consumers. Some freeing up of these restrictions, it was felt, was necessary to facilitate consumer access to a wide variety of healthcare professionals and to help contain healthcare costs.[92] For instance, certain services being provided by physicians or dentists could be performed by competent, but less highly trained (and less costly) practitioners, such as physician assistants or dental hygienists.

Medical professionals and state licensure boards opposed the provision, arguing that more permissive practice laws would jeopardize the quality of care being delivered and that the federal government would be encroaching into a field of regulation more properly left to the states. However, the proposed amendment did generate some support from consumer-based organizations. For instance, in a February 1994 statement to Congress, the Citizen Advocacy Center called the amendment "one of the golden rules of licensure in the public interest." But by fall 1994, the federal preemption provision met the same fate as the Health Security Act that encompassed it.[93]

Providing Federal Grants to State Medical Boards

With much the same consumer-protection rationale as Congressman Stark had for proposing his federal mandate for physician recredentialing, Congressman Wyden offered an initiative to provide federal financial support to state medical boards. He, too, felt that in itself the National Practitioner Data Bank failed to provide sufficient protection against incompetent physicians and that state medical boards were insufficiently responsive to this danger.

Compared with the above two failed proposals, Wyden's proposal was more deferential to the state boards. In his amendment to the Health Security Act in the spring of 1994, he called for the provision of federal grants-in-aid to state medical boards meeting certain prescribed federal performance standards.[94] Among the standards specified were those requiring that: (1) nonphysicians account for at least 51 percent of the members of the boards; (2) all licensure fees imposed by the states on physicians be used to support the activities of the boards; and (3) boards investigate any "credible evidence" alleging physician incompetence. Wyden knew the first standard would be unpopular with medical professionals, but the other standards were reasonably nonthreatening. Notably absent were any standards addressing state recredentialing or scope-of-practice laws.

Adding further to the political feasibility of the measure was that it built on a prior proposal introduced by President Bush as part of a medical malpractice reform package. That package, never enacted, included a series of tort reforms.[95] But it also included—as a quid pro quo—a provision intended to support state medical board efforts to identify and discipline physicians practicing substandard medicine. The provision, cosponsored by subsequent Speaker of the House Newt Gingrich among others, was to provide financial grants to state boards, albeit without the kinds of performance standards now being proposed by Wyden.

A coalition of more than 25 consumer groups supported the Wyden measure. In a statement directed to the President and Congress, the coalition warned, "Please do not miss this opportunity to design a consumer-focused system or you will be hearing from your constituents when the system fails."[96] Among state licensure boards and healthcare professionals, the Wyden proposal, while not as threatening as the others, still represented federal encroachment that was unsettling.[97] In the heat of the battle over healthcare reform, it was a minor issue and faded away without much notice.

Conclusion

Why did the above three initiatives fail to pass? The basic answer is that the sense of peril was insufficient to counter the federal government's deep-seated bias toward inaction. Neither cost-containment nor consumer protection rationales were sufficiently present or compelling to enable enactment. In our political system, this is the fate of the great majority of federal initiatives proposed to regulate healthcare professionals.

But it would be misleading simply to dismiss these initiatives as failures. After all, their sponsors succeeded in getting them on the political agenda.[98] The measures drew some attention to concerns that may not be adequately addressed by the states, the professions, or the private market and that may yet intensify. And they advanced approaches to confronting these concerns that may yet emerge as the bases for federal action.[99]

In this context, a federal regulatory initiative that may lack sufficient backing in itself could still become enacted if it were part of a larger package that includes provisions attractive to the professions. The National Practitioner Data Bank, as we have seen, emerged as an idea in good currency in 1984 when the GAO drew attention to disciplined physicians moving from one state to another, but did not become law until a few years later when it was packaged in a bill affording the medical profession peer review protections it sought.

Our review suggests that federal efforts to regulate healthcare professionals that are not part of some such quid pro quo may have little prospect of enactment unless cost containment is an overriding factor. This was the case with the two enacted federal initiatives examined above that were not packaged with other features offering significant inducements to professional interests. Both the Medicare PSRO/PRO legislation and the Medicaid DUR legislation were passed in response to pressing concerns about escalating program costs and clear congressional expectations to achieve savings. Consumer protection concerns and expectations were part of the mix, but were of distinctly secondary concern.

Our review also suggests that what professionals cannot achieve at the time of program enactment, may become attainable during program implementation. In this process, professionals, because of their expertise and political influence, exert continuing influence in ways that bias the efforts toward their own interests, with little countervailing influence by consumer-based interests. This is evident in the transformation of the PRO program, which at this point functions very much as an extension of a professional association, seeking to elevate the practice of medicine, but disinclined to use its authorities to protect the public from incompetent practitioners. Similarly, the DUR program has evolved in a way that exerts little muscle against physicians or pharmacists responsible for poor prescribing or dispensing practices.

Thus, federal initiatives to regulate healthcare professionals, even in those rare cases when they become enacted, may not be as threatening as professionals fear or as influential as consumers and taxpayers may hope. The process of carrying out the initiatives does not occur in neutral political space, but in environments where professionals have ample opportunities to mold the initiatives in ways and toward ends they find more acceptable than those spelled out in the originating legislation.

In 1994, the demise of the Clinton health plan marked the end of a major governmental effort to reform healthcare financing and delivery on a national scale. But it also was accompanied by the acceleration of market-driven reforms that have proven to be no less sweeping. Traditional fee-for-service medical practice has been rapidly giving way to managed care arrangements under which HMOs and physicians share financial risk.[100] Further, in the quest to maximize their financial advantage in an environment with heightened price sensitivity, hospitals, HMOs, and physician groups have been engaged in far-reaching consolidations (with one another and separately) that have given rise to huge, powerful healthcare corporations dominating the healthcare marketplace.[101]

Business managers, drawing on their corporations' market leverage and healthcare research's success in producing medical practice guidelines, exert more control than ever over practicing professionals.[102] Patients, even those that are beneficiaries of federal programs, find that they are expected to act as informed buyers in a marketplace. Medical professionals find that in many respects they become middlemen, aiming to satisfy both the organizations with which they are affiliated and the patients they serve. They face conflicting obligations to a business ethic and to their long-standing service ethic.[103]

Although government has not been the architect of the market-based reforms, it has increasingly been inclined to shape its own policies in response to them. This is quite apparent in the Medicare and Medicaid programs, where both the federal and state governments have been taking on a business orientation, seeking to act as prudent purchasers of healthcare services on behalf of their customers—Medicare and Medicaid beneficiaries.[104] Along this line, both programs have been looking to managed care for cost savings and have been contracting widely with HMOs toward this end.[105]

In the public-private partnerships that have been evolving, the HMOs have been regulating the practice of healthcare professionals to a degree that federal policymakers could not possibly gain the political support to do directly. To contain costs and ensure healthcare of appropriate quality, HMOs are checking the credentials of professionals affiliated with them, defining acceptable parameters of their practice, collecting data that document their practice patterns and how they compare with one another, and determining what if any corrective actions to take against them if they are found to be practicing in unacceptable ways.

In this highly commercialized environment, dominated by a number of large, proprietary HMOs, significant pressures have been building for governmental regulation that helps protect professionals and consumers from the excesses (real or perceived) of the marketplace. For some time, the AMA has been advocating "patient protection" legislation that would help preserve physicians' clinical independence and patients' right to chose physicians of their choice. Physician and consumer interests have been joining forces to support legislation that would prohibit practices such as health plan "gag clauses" that impede physician-patient communication or "drive-through deliveries" that take place because of health plan policies limiting hospital stays for women giving birth. In September 1996, the President signed into law a bill that guarantees mothers and their infants coverage for a 48-hour hospital stay for normal births.[106]

Thus far, these recent pressures for regulation have been exerted and addressed primarily at the state level. But their presence at the federal level has also been quite apparent. Many bills have been introduced in Congress to protect patients against various HMO practices. Indeed, at the 1996 Democratic national convention, both the President and First Lady made clear in their official remarks that they supported federal legislation that would preclude HMOs from requiring mothers and their babies to leave hospitals less than 48 hours after delivery.[107]

The managed care industry has been strongly opposed to regulatory efforts (whether at state or federal levels) that seek to constrain their leverage over healthcare professionals. But as much as it may be opposed to governmental regulation, when regulation does occur or seems inevitable, the industry may well be more receptive to federal than to state regulation. In an industry that is increasingly consolidated across state lines, it is much more efficient for it to work with one set of national rules than 50 sets of state rules. Imagine the inefficiencies the industry would confront, for example, if it had to interact with 50 state practitioner data banks rather than one national one.

This is not to suggest that further federal regulation of healthcare professionals is inevitable in the years ahead. Radio talk shows, newspaper exposes, and books such as P. J. O'Rourke's *Parliament of Whores* both reflect and help to sustain a deep-seated skepticism about government in general and the federal government in particular.[108] This popular mood could yet lead Congress to scale back or even eliminate any or all of the enacted federal initiatives discussed in this chapter.

Yet there are significant forces at work that could lead to further federal regulation. The most obvious perhaps are those that limit the controls exerted by HMOs. But other perhaps more imposing forces also warrant attention in this regard. Concerns about the perilous state of the Medicare trust fund could well trigger some forceful federal actions that have consequences for professional practice. So too could concerns about the vulnerabilities faced by the many millions of people in the country who remain medically uninsured.

In this climate, the tide of federal initiatives to regulate healthcare professionals will continue to ebb and flow. But given the forces noted above, it is quite possible that in the near future there will be more flow than ebb.

Notes

1. A. Koch and W. Peden (eds.). 1944. *The Life and Selected Writings of Thomas Jefferson*. New York: Random House.

2. M. R. Haug and M. B. Sussman. 1969. "Professional Autonomy and the Revolt of the Client. *Social Problems* 17 (2): 153–61; H. L. Wilensky. 1964. "The Professionalization of Everyone?" *American Journal of Sociology* 70 (2): 137–58; R. H. Hall. 1968. "Professionalization and Bureaucratization." *American Sociological Review* (February): 92–104; D. Blumenthal. 1994. "The Vital Role of Professionalism in Health Care Reform." *Health Affairs* 13 (1): 252–56.

3. This rationale, it should be noted, centers on providing consumers with certain minimum protections. It should be distinguished from efforts that seek continuous improvements in the process or outcomes of professional practice (which is the focus of the quality assurance programs of most healthcare institutions today). T. L. Jost. 1995. "Oversight of the Quality of Medical Care: Regulation, Management, or the Market?" *Arizona Law Review* 37 (3): 825–68.

4. This legislation indicates how the desire to increase access to healthcare services can also be an important force affecting the regulation of healthcare professionals. In

this instance, the congressional intent to increase access established a programmatic infrastructure that inevitably led to various regulations directed to professionals participating in these programs. As we will see, cost and consumer protection concerns were influential in shaping some of the most prominent of these regulations.

5. See J. K. Iglehart. 1992. "The American Health Care System: Medicare." *New England Journal of Medicine* 327 (20): 1467–72; and J. K. Iglehart. 1993. "Health Policy Report: Medicaid." *New England Journal of Medicine* 328 (12): 896–900.

6. The Medicare and Medicaid programs have been central forces driving the federal role in regulating healthcare professionals. The federal interest in cost containment, for instance, has been largely defined by these two programs. Also of note is that specific regulatory initiatives that extend beyond these programs often have used either or both of them as the "hook" for imposing federal influence over the states or professions.

7. U.S. General Accounting Office. 1972. "Problems with Evaluating the Cost-Effectiveness of Professional Standards Review Organizations." July; Congressional Budget Office. 1981. "The Effect of PSROs on Health Care Costs: Current Findings and Future Evaluations." June; Congressional Budget Office. 1981. "The Impact of PSROs on Health Care Costs: Update of CBO's 1979 Evaluation." January.

8. Unlike the grant-funded PSROs, the PROs had fixed-price contracts with measurable performance objectives (42 U.S.C. 1320c-2).

9. Created by the Tax Equity and Fiscal Responsibility Act of 1982 (P.L. 97-248).

10. U.S. Congress. Senate. Committee on Finance, Subcommittee on Health. *Hearings on Proposals to Make Improvements in Professional Standards Review Organizations.* 97th Cong., 2nd sess., 1982.

11. Once patients' diagnoses were determined, Medicare would pay hospitals a fixed amount regardless of the costs incurred by the hospital. The Social Security Amendments of 1983 (P.L. 98-21). See D. G. Smith. 1992. *Paying for Medicare: The Politics of Reform.* New York: Aldine De Gruyter.

12. Consolidated Omnibus Budget Reconciliation Act of 1985 (P.L. 99-272). 42 U.S.C. 1320c-3(a)(2). Final regulations to implement this provision have never been issued.

13. The Omnibus Reconciliation Act of 1986 (P.L. 99-509).

14. U.S. Congress. Senate. Committee on Finance. *Hearings on the Examination of Quality of Care Under Medicare's Prospective Payment System.* 99th Cong., 2nd sess., 1986.

15. HHS/OIG. 1988. "Quality Review Activities." HHS/OIG. 1988. "Sanction Activities"; HHS/OIG. 1989. "The Utilization and Quality Control Peer Review Organization Program: A Review of Program Effectiveness."

16. HHS. Health Care Financing Administration. Request for Proposals and Scope of Work, 1988.

17. U.S. Congress. House. Committee on Ways and Means. *Hearings on the Medicare Peer Review Organization Program.* 104th Cong., 1st sess., 1995.

18. HHS/OIG. 1992. "Educating Physicians Responsible for Poor Care: A Review of the Peer Review Organizations' Efforts."

19. Citizen Advocacy Center (CAC). 1992. "Information Exchange Between Peer

Review Organizations and Medical Licensing Boards. Report on the 50 State Survey." March; CAC. 1992. "Update and Report on CAC Survey." November; HHS/OIG. 1993. "The Peer Review Organizations and State Medical Boards: A Vital Link." April.

20. From 1986 through 1995, PROs referred a total of 285 physicians and providers to the OIG for sanction. Most referrals occurred in the earliest years of the program: 66 in fiscal year (FY) 1986, 72 in FY 1987, and 37 in FY 1988. In FYs 1991 through 1994, PRO referrals hovered between 12 and 14 per year. In FY 1995, the PROs referred just seven. (Office of Investigations. Office of Inspector General. U.S. Department of Health and Human Services.)

21. D. E. Berwick. 1989. "Continuous Quality Improvement as an Ideal in Health Care." *New England Journal of Medicine* 320 (1): 53; Jost, 1995, "Oversight of the Quality of Medical Care: Regulation, Management, or the Market?"

22. IOM. 1990. *Medicare: A Strategy for Quality Assurance.*

23. S. F. Jencks and G. R. Wilensky. 1992. "The Health Care Quality Improvement Initiative: A New Approach to Quality Assurance in Medicare." *Journal of the American Medical Association* 269 (7): 900.

24. B. Gagel, quoted in "HCFA Blasts PRO Performance." *Utilization Review* (21 January 1993).

25. Jencks and Wilensky, "The Health Care Quality Improvement Initiative."

26. "Congress gave HCFA its blessing to move the program in a new direction. . . . All this stuff was done by administrative edict." Andy Webber, quoted in R. C. Cunningham (ed.). 1996. "Cops or Colleagues? Fuzzy Standards for Judging PROs." *Medicine & Health* (13 May): 1–4.

27. U.S. Congress. House. Committee on Ways and Means. *Hearings on the Medicare Peer Review Organization Program.* 104th Cong., 1st sess., 1995.

28. HHS/OIG. 1995. "The Medicare Peer Review Organizations' Role in Identifying and Responding to Poor Performers." See also L. O. Praeger. 1996. "Inspector General: Can PROs Effectively Teach and Police?" *American Medical News* 39 (9): 3, 30.

29. GAO. 1996. "Medicare: Federal Efforts to Enhance Patient Quality of Care."

30. Cunningham (ed.), "Cops or Colleagues?"

31. On June 5, 1996, the Medicare Trustees reported that the hospital insurance trust fund will be depleted by the year 2001. (HHS Press Release, 5 June 1996.)

32. As of August 1996, 10.2 percent of Medicare beneficiaries were enrolled in risk-sharing managed care organizations—almost twice as many as were enrolled five years before. (U.S. Department of Health and Human Services, Health Care Financing Administration.)

33. Following are some recent stories prominently reported in the media: "Florida Doctor Sanctioned in New Amputation." *The Boston Globe*, 19 July 1995; "Unlicensed Surgeon Targeted by Maryland: Officials Say Doctor Failed a Dozen Exams." *The Washington Post*, 5 October 1995; "State Issues Scathing Report on Error at Sloan-Kettering." *The New York Times*, 16 November 1995; "Overdoses Still Weigh Heavily at Dana-Farber." *The Boston Globe*, 26 December 1995; "Surgeon Accused of Conspiring to Violate Drug-Safety Rules." *The New York Times*, 18 January 1996; "Most Doctors with Violations Keep Their License."

The New York Times, 29 March 1996; R. Saltus. 1996. "Two Surgeons Surrender Licenses after Mistakenly Removing Kidney." *The Boston Globe*, 6 June.

34. E. E. Lipowski and T. Collins. 1995. *Medicaid DUR Programs: 1993*. Washington, DC: American Pharmaceutical Association Foundation; T. R. Fulda and S. L. Hass. 1992. "Medicaid Drug Utilization Review under OBRA 1990: Current Issues and Future Directions." *PharmacoEconomics* 2 (5): 363–64 1, U.S. Congress. Senate. Special Committee on Aging. *The Cost-Effectiveness of Drug Utilization Review: An Annotated Bibliography*, 101st Cong., 2nd sess., October 1990.

35. S. W. Kidder. 1987. "The Cost-Benefit of Pharmacist-Conducted Drug Regimen Reviews." *The Consultant Pharmacist* (September/October): 398.

36. The Medicare DUR program was a component of the Medicare Catastrophic Coverage Act that Congress passed in June 1988 and then repealed in November 1989 in response to widespread protests among the elderly over the costs that the legislation would impose on them.

37. The Omnibus Budget Reconciliation Act of 1990 (P.L. 101-508).

38. See Fulda and Hass, "Medicaid Drug Utilization Review under OBRA 1990," 363–65.

39. See Special Committee on Aging, *The Cost-Effectiveness of Drug Utilization Review*, Foreword.

40. 42 U.S.C. 1396r-8.

41. See AMA. 1990. "Drug Utilization Review." *Board of Trustees Report R*, adopted by House of Delegates, December; see also AMA. 1992. *Statement to the Health Care Financing Administration on Medicaid Drug Use Review Program*, 9 December.

42. H. A. Smith. 1992. "Drug Utilization Review and the New Medicaid Requirements." *Journal of Pharmacoepidemiology* 2 (4): 53–71; G. Borzo. 1994. "Mandated Drug Review Expands Role of Pharmacists." *American Medical News* (17 January); 1, 30, 35. In response to pharmacist concerns about reimbursement for counseling services, the legislation called for a demonstration project on the cost effectiveness of reimbursement for pharmacists' cognitive services.

43. 42 C.F.R. 456. Also, Health Care Financing Administration, Memorandum to Medicaid DUR Coordinators. 1994. "DUR Annual Report Instructions for FFY 1994." 3 February.

44. HHS. Health Care Financing Administration. 1995. "Medicare and Medicaid Statistical Supplement." *Health Care Financing Review* (February): 362.

45. Lipowski and Collins, *Medicaid DUR Programs*, 14.

46. HHS/OIG. 1995. *Medicaid Drug Use Review Programs: Lessons Learned by States* (May): 25; Lipowski and Collins, *Medicaid DUR Programs*, 15–16; W. J. Moore. 1994. "Medicaid Drug Utilization Review: A Critical Appraisal." *Medical Care Review* 51 (1): 3–37.

47. For pharmacists, this irritation has been attenuated by the fact that the Federal legislation led many states to modify their state pharmacy acts to call for drug utilization review as part of the practice of pharmacy. These modifications serve to reinforce the pharmacist's role as a professional caregiver. Often states have incorporated problem definitions into their computerized claims-screening criteria causing many false positives, with the result that much pharmacist and even physician time is taken up addressing prescriptions that are properly written. See

HHS/OIG, *Medicaid Drug Use Review Programs*, 8–9. For a review of the benefits of the pro-DUR systems, see, GAO. 1996. *Prescription Drugs and Medicaid: Automated Systems Can Help Promote Safety, Save Money.* (11 June).

48. These criteria are usually part of a proprietary set of criteria used by vendors in different settings. See HHS/OIG, *Medicaid Drug Use Review Programs*, 24.

49. Note the following opening line of a health information newsletter: "Drug utilization review (UR) is the opening of another front in the battle against rising health costs." C. Kent (ed.). 1992. "Drug Utilization Review: Apocalypse When?" *Medicine and Health* (24 February).

50. Lipowski and Collins, *Medicaid DUR Programs*, 2. Also, earlier, a member of that team warned that the lack of adequate research on the effects of DUR might inhibit its potential, with the result that "DUR efforts may be limited to cost-containment issues without due consideration of quality-of-care outcomes." (H. L. Lipton. 1993. "Drug Utilization Review in Ambulatory Settings: State of the Scene and Directions for Outcome Research." *Medical Care* 31 (12): 1069.)

51. HHS/OIG, *Medicaid Drug Use Review Programs.*

52. L. Etheredge. 1995. *Pharmacy Benefit Management: The Right RX?* Research Agenda Brief. Washington, DC: George Washington University, April.

53. HHS/OIG. 1996. *Medicaid Drug Use Review Programs*, 26. See also, "Quick Change: More Medicaid Programs Turning to Managed Care." *Drug Topics* (8 April): 78–79.

54. GAO. 1984. *Expanded Federal Authority Needed to Protect Medicare and Medicaid Patients From Health Practitioners Who Lose Their Licenses.* (1 May).

55. In the Senate, the hearings were before the U.S. Senate Special Committee on Aging. In the House, they were before the Subcommittee on Health of the Committee on Ways and Means and the Subcommittee on Health of the Committee on Energy and Commerce. The legislation introduced in the 98th Congress, 2nd Session was entitled the "Medicare and Medicaid Patient and Program Protection Act of 1984"—H.R. 5989 and S. 2744.

56. Similar legislation was introduced in 1985. See U.S. Congress. House. Committee on Ways and Means, Subcommittee on Health and the Environment. *Hearings on Medicare and Medicaid Patient and Program Protection Act.* 99th Cong., 1st sess., 1985.

57. At about the same time that the GAO issued its final report, the *Detroit Free Press* was running a seven-part series entitled: "Bad Doctors/License to Err?" (D. Katz. 1984. *Detroit Free Press*, 1–8 April). In the fall of 1985, the *New York Times* ran two stories on medical incompetence, the second of which ran under the heading: "Medical Discipline Laws: Confusion Reigns" (J. Brinkley. 1985. *The New York Times*, 3 September). The *Boston Globe*, during the following summer, ran a five-part series on the "Malpractice Malady" (*The Boston Globe*, June 1986).

58. HHS/OIG. 1986. *Medical Licensure and Discipline: An Overview.* (June). This report was followed by similar OIG reports concerning other state licensure authorities: *State Licensure and Discipline of Dentists* (August 1988); *State Licensure and Discipline of Podiatrists* (December 1988); *State Licensure and Discipline of Chiropractors* (January 1989); and *State Licensure and Discipline of Optometrists* (February 1989).

59. For example, A. Gellhorn et al. 1984. New York State Department of Health. *Report*

of the Committee on Medical Credentials (27 June); Office of the Auditor General of California. 1985. *The State's Diversion Programs Do Not Adequately Protect the Public from Health Professionals Who Suffer from Alcoholism or Drug Abuse* (January); Joint Committee of the New Jersey State Board of Higher Education and the New Jersey State Board of Medical Examiners. 1987. *Strengthening Educational and Licensure Standards for Physicians in New Jersey*, Volume One (March).

60. *Patrick v. Burget*, 486 U.S. 94 (1988). The judgment was subsequently reversed by the Federal Court of Appeals for the Ninth Circuit and then reaffirmed by the United States Supreme Court. See *Patrick v. Burget*, 800 F. 2d 1498 (9th Cir. 1986), and *Patrick v. Burget*, 486 U.S. 94, at 94.

61. J. K. Iglehart. 1987. "Congress Moves to Bolster Peer Review: The Health Care Quality Improvement Act of 1986." *New England Journal of Medicine* 316 (15): 960–64; H. A. Waxman. 1987. "Medical Malpractice and Quality of Care." *New England Journal of Medicine* 316 (15): 943–44.

62. U.S. Congress. House. Committee on Energy and Commerce, Subcommittee on Health and the Environment. *Hearing on H.R. 5110, The Health Care Quality Improvement Act of 1986.* 99th Cong., 2nd sess., 1986.

63. P.L. 99-660. In the first statement of congressional findings at the beginning of the Title, Congress specified that the legislation was responding to "nationwide problems that warrant greater efforts than those that can be achieved by any individual state."

64. A year later, Congressman Wyden spearheaded the passage of follow-up legislation, the Medicare and Medicaid Patient Protection Act of 1987. This legislation extended federal exclusionary authority along the lines called for in the proposed 1984 legislation. It also called for disciplinary actions taken against other types of healthcare practitioners to be reported to a national repository. As of this writing, there have been no appropriations made to support this requirement, and it has not yet been implemented. However, in August 1996, as part of the "Health Insurance Portability and Accountability Act of 1996" (P.L. 104-91), Congress authorized a new adverse action data bank for the reporting of final adverse actions against healthcare practitioners. How this would relate to the National Practitioner Data Bank and the reporting called for in the 1987 legislation remain to be determined as of this writing.

65. Both the AMA and the Federation of State Medical Boards considered submitting bids as the data bank contractor. But they soon lost interest as they became aware of HHS expectations and HHS disinclination to work with them.

66. R. Scalettar. 1986. *Statement of the American Medical Association to the Subcommittee on Health and the Environment, Committee on Energy and Commerce, U.S. House of Representatives, Re the Quality of Medical Care and Physician Discipline*, 15 July, 10.

67. GAO. 1990. *National Health Practitioner Data Bank Has Not Been Well Managed.* (August).

68. M. Holoweiko. 1991. "The Malpractice Data Bank is Turning into a Frankenstein." *Medical Economics* 68 (6 May): 120–33.

69. J. Lapinski. 1992. "National Practioner Data Bank—Incomplete and Future Cloudy." *Physician Executive* 18 (2): 28–33.

70. GAO. 1983. *National Practitioner Data Bank Continues to Experience Problems.* (January): 2.

71. P. A. Ross. 1992. "The National Practitioner Data Bank." *Health Systems REVIEW*

(September/October): 44–46.

72. L. Corbin. 1993. "Excellence in Technology: 1993 Federal Leadership Awards." *Government Executive* (November): 35–36.

73. HHS/OIG. 1995. *National Practitioner Data Bank Reports to Hospitals: Their Usefulness and Impact.* (April); R. E. Oshel, T. Croft, and J. Rodak. 1995. "The National Practitioner Data Bank." *Public Health Reports* 110 (4): 383–94; M. R. Yessian. 1995. "Putting the Controversy Aside, How Is the Data Bank Doing?" *Public Health Reports* 110 (4): 381–82.

74. M. Pretzer. 1994. "Is The Malpractice Data Bank Going Public?" *Medical Economics* 71 (26 September): 81.

75. In 1995, the AMA House of Delegates resolved that AMA policy 355.987, "calling for the dissolution of the National Practitioner Data Bank, be reaffirmed. . . ."

76. For an indication of the nature of organized dentistry's concerns about how the Data Bank would impede professional self-regulation, see J. L. Shub. 1991. "National Practitioner Data Bank: Understanding Its Debits and Credits." *New York State Dental Journal* (January): 31–34.

77. HHS/OIG. 1993. "National Practitioner Data Bank: Usefulness and Impact of Reports to Hospitals" (February); HHS/OIG. 1995. "National Practitioner Data Bank Reports to Hospitals" (February); HHS/OIG. 1995. "National Practitioner Data Bank Reports to Managed Care Organizations: Their Usefulness and Impact" (April); HHS/OIG. 1984. "National Practitioner Data Bank: Profile of Matches Update" (August).

78. See "Comments on the Draft Report," in HHS/OIG. *National Practitioner Data Bank Reports to Hospitals.* See also, J. S. Todd. 1983. "National Practitioner Data Bank: Worthy of Consumer Confidence?" *Federation Bulletin* 80 (4): 226–30; J. S. Todd. 1995. "Just Numbers or Knowledge?" *Public Health Reports* 110 (4): 377–78.

79. The legislation was introduced as H.R. 4274, Health Care Quality Improvement Act Amendments of 1994.

80. "CAC Supports Proposed Amendments to the National Practitioner Data Bank Legislation." *Citizen Advocacy News* (Newsletter of the Citizen Advocacy Center), 2nd Quarter, 1994; See also S. M. Wolfe. 1993. "The Need for Public Access to the National Practitioner Data Bank." *Federation Bulletin* 80 (4): 231–35; S. M. Wolfe. 1995. "Congress Should Open the National Practitioner Data Bank to All." *Public Health Reports* 110 (4): 378–79.

81. J. Brinkley. 1994. "You Bet Your Life: Do You Know the Odds?" *The New York Times,* 29 May.

82. HHS, Health Resources and Services Administration, Bureau of Health Professions, Division of Quality Assurance. The AMA tends to discount the significant increase in voluntary queries by managed care organizations, suggesting that these are attributable to national accreditation requirements. Todd, "Just Numbers or Knowledge," 377. Yet, it still holds that the accrediting body must find the data bank to be conducive to effective credentials verification if it mandates that managed care organizations receiving accreditation regularly query the data bank.

83. "A Survey of the Future of Medicine." *Economist* 330 (19 March 1994): 1–18.

84. Press Release 24, "The Honorable Pete Stark (D. Calif.), Chairman, Subcommittee

on Health, Committee on Ways and Means, U.S. House of Representatives, Announces a Hearing on Physician Recertification." 29 March 1990.

85. The bill was introduced as H.R. 4464, The Medicare Physician Qualification Act of 1990. It gave the HHS Secretary the authority to determine qualified examinations and to approve state licensure programs. The penalty for physicians failing to qualify was that they could not be reimbursed for services under the Medicare program.

86. Early the following year, the *Journal of the American Medical Association* published both an article and an editorial concerning the New York plans. See A. G. Gellhorn. 1991. "Periodic Physician Recredentialing." *Journal of the American Medical Association* 265 (6): 752–55; D. G. Langsley. 1991. "Recredentialing." *Journal of the American Medical Association* 265 (6): 772.

87. *Citizen Advocacy News*, 1st Quarter, 1994.

88. U.S. Congress. House. Committee on Ways and Means, Subcommittee on Health. *Hearing on Physician Recertification*. 101st Cong., 2nd sess., 1990.

89. U.S. Congress. House. Committee on Ways and Means, Subcommittee on Health. *Hearings Regarding HR 4464: Periodic Recertification of Physicians*. 101st Cong., 2nd sess., 1990. The Federation of State Medical Boards also testified against the proposed legislation. The federation's executive director indicated that it would be better to rely on stronger mandatory reporting requirements to "steadily improve identification of unqualified, unfit, and impaired physicians." See *Citizen Advocacy News*, 1st Quarter, 1994.

90. See S. Steinmo and J. Watts. 1995. "It's the Institutions, Stupid! Why Comprehensive National Health Insurance Always Fails in America." *Journal of Health Politics, Policy and Law* 20 (2): 329–72. This issue includes a "Roundtable on the Defeat of Reform" that offers a wide range of explanations for the demise of the Clinton health plan. See also T. Skocpol. 1995. "The Rise and Resounding Demise of the Clinton Plan." *Health Affairs* 14 (1): 66–85.

91. Section 1161 of H.R. 3600.

92. National Council of State Boards of Nursing. 1993. *Federal Preemption of State Licensing: A Review Paper Prepared by Vedder, Price, Kaufman & Kammholz* (December); *Citizen Advocacy News*, 1st Quarter, 1994.

93. The staying power of reforming state healthcare licensure laws was reaffirmed about a year later when the Pew Health Professions Commission came out with a report calling for extensive reform in healthcare workforce regulation. It criticized state licensure laws for providing "broad, near-exclusive scopes of practice to a few professions and 'carved out' scopes for the remaining professions"; such laws, it warned, "erect unreasonable barriers to high quality and affordable care." Yet, well aware of the political tenor of the times and of the fate of recent federal initiatives to challenge state regulatory authority, the Pew Commission steered away from any call for federal action and directed its many proposed reforms to state governments. (Pew Health Professions Commission. *Reforming Health Care Workforce Regulation: Policy Considerations for the 21st Century*. Report of the Task Force on Health Care Workforce Regulation (December 1995): vii; see also L. O. Praeger. 1995. "Licensing Proposals Seek to Overhaul Current System." *American Medical News* (2 October): 6.)

94. Section 5013 of H.R. 3600.

95. These provisions were reflected in S. 489 and H.R. 1004 introduced in 1991, during

the first session of the 102nd Congress. The President proposed his malpractice reform initiative as the Health Care Liability Reform and Quality of Care Improvement Act of 1991. It was announced in a White House press release on May 15, 1991. For a newspaper report, see P. J. Hilts. 1991. "Bush Enters Malpractice Debate with Plan to Limit Court Awards." *The New York Times*, 13 May.

96. Coalition for Consumer Protection and Quality in Health Care Reform, *Testimony Before the Subcommittee on Health for Families and the Uninsured, Committee on Finance, United Sates Senate.* (29 April 1994).

97. Indicative of the congressional concern about federal encroachment is the fact that many in Congress were expressing unease with the Republican-initiated malpractice reforms because "they would curtail states' rights to determine their own approach to the problems." See Hilts, "Bush Enters Malpractice Debate." (13 May).

98. D. A. Rochefort and R. W. Cobb (eds.). 1994. *The Politics of Problem Definition: Shaping the Policy Agenda*. Lawrence, KS: University Press of Kansas.

99. Donald Schon has described this process as one involving the emergence of "ideas in good currency." See D. A. Schon. 1973. *Beyond the Stable State*. New York: W. W. Norton and Co.

100. For a thorough review of these trends, see Prospective Payment Assessment Commission. *Medicare and the American Health Care System: Report to Congress* (June 1996).

101. M. Freudenheim. 1996. "Managed Care Empires in the Making: Companies Build Networks to Stay Ahead of a Hard-Charging Field." *The New York Times*, 2 April, D 1; J. Johnsson. 1996. "Insurer-HMO Mega Merger." *American Medical News* (4 April): 1, 23; C. Tokarski. 1996. "Huge Merger Aims for East Coast: NJ Blues Consolidation Leaves Local Doctors Edgy." *American Medical News* (17 June): 1, 30–31.

102. J. A. Morone and G. S. Belkin. "The Science Illusion and the Triumph of Medical Capitalism." Paper delivered at the 1995 Annual Meeting of the American Political Science Association. Chicago, IL (31 August–2 September 1995).

103. E. Ginzburg. 1995. "A Cautionary Note on Market Reforms in Health Care." *Journal of the American Medical Association* 274 (20): 1633–34; S. Woolhandler and D. U. Himmelstein. 1995. "Extreme Risk—The New Corporate Proposition for Physicians." *New England Journal of Medicine* 333 (25): 1706–7; P. B. Ginsburg and J. M. Grossman. 1995. "Health System Change: The View from Wall Street." *Health Affairs* 14 (4): 159–63; J. Somerville. 1996. "Medicaid HMO Market Fight: The Risks of Profit." *American Medical News* 39 (15): 3, 29–30.

104. L. Etheredge. *Reengineering Medicare: From Bill-Paying Insurer to Accountable Purchaser*. Research Agenda Brief. (Washington, DC: George Washington University, June 1995); S. Jones and L. Etheredge. *Paradigm Shifts in Medicare Reform*. Research Agenda Brief. (Washington, DC: George Washington University, April 1996); D. Rowland and K. Hanson. 1996. "Medicaid: Moving to Managed Care." *Health Affairs* 15 (3): 150–52.

105. The Health Care Financing Administration in the U.S. Department of Health and Human Services reports that, as of August 1996, 10.2 percent of Medicare beneficiaries were enrolled in risk-sharing HMOs. It did not have available a comparable compilation for Medicaid beneficiaries. As of this writing, HCFA's most recent data on Medicaid managed care enrollment date from June 30, 1996. They indicate that, as of that time, 39 percent of Medicaid beneficiaries were in managed

care arrangements. However, many, and perhaps most of these beneficiaries, were not enrolled in HMOs, but rather in primary care case management plans that call for them to access medical care through primary care physicians.

106. C. Kent. 1995. "Bill Would Put the Brakes on 'Drive-Through Deliveries.'" *American Medical News* (2 October): 1, 19; R. Kreier. 1995. "N.Y. Suit Fights Increasingly Common HMO 'Gag Rules'" *American Medical News* (11 December): 5, 7; S. S. Hsu. 1996. "Va. Assembly Begins Writing Prescription for Medical Care: Intense Fight Opens over Shape of Health Plans." *Washington Post*, 18 March; M. Freudenheim. 1996. "HMOs Cope with a Backlash on Cost-Cutting." *The New York Times*, 19 May; R. Cunningham (ed.). 1996. "Backlash: How Worried Should Health Plans Be?" *Medicine and Health* (3 June); Families USA Foundation, *HMO Consumers at Risk: States to the Rescue* (July 1996). D. Gianelli. 1996. "Mandating Coverage." *American Medical News* (14 October): 1, 25.

107. It is also of note in this context that the AMA has been advocating for federal legislation that would facilitate the establishment of physician-run organizations that operate independently of HMOs and toward that end would allow for federal preemption of state licensing requirements in cases where the latter proved to be obstructive. Such legislation was incorporated as Section 1854 in the proposed Medicare Preservation Act of 1995 (H.R. 2485). The proposed legislation was not passed.

108. P. J. O'Rourke. 1991. *Parliament of Whores: A Lone Humorist Attempts to Explore the Entire U.S. Government.* New York: Atlantic Monthly Press. It is also pertinent to note here that the proportion of the American public indicating that "most of the time" it could trust "the government in Washington to do what is right," dropped from 57 percent in 1958 to 20 percent in 1993. See B. W. Roper. 1994. "Democracy in America: How Are We Doing?" *The Public Perspective* 5 (3): 3.

REGULATION OF THE MEDICAL PROFESSION: A PHYSICIAN'S PERSPECTIVE

Arnold S. Relman

THIS CHAPTER reflects on many of the issues discussed in this book. The perspective is that of a physician who has been a clinical practitioner and consultant, a medical educator and administrator, a member of a specialty certifying board, the editor of a general medical journal, and, during the past few years, a member of a state medical board. The views expressed here are entirely the author's own, based on this experience. They do not necessarily reflect the position of any of the organizations with which he has been, or is now, associated.

General Considerations

This commentary begins with the proposition that physicians have a social contract with the state. They are licensed by the state to practice medicine, thereby gaining considerable power and authority over the delivery of medical services and, as a consequence, receiving substantial material advantages. In exchange, physicians make a commitment to serve the medical needs of their patients, with diligence, competence, and integrity. This fiduciary commitment takes precedence over considerations of private gain and personal convenience. State boards control licensure, but they expect the profession to share responsibility for its own regulation and discipline. Deferring to professional expertise, boards usually look to the profession to set the standards for education and specialty certification. The profession is also expected, through various kinds of peer review and quality assurance procedures based mainly in hospitals and clinics, to monitor the competence of its members, and to identify and correct most problems in these spheres. However, physicians must be accountable to the state licensing boards and be prepared to demonstrate that they are meeting their commitment. Licenses, once conferred, do not guarantee life-long professional competence and integrity. Since the state holds the authority to license, the boards are ultimately responsible for protecting the public against unethical and incompetent practitioners, and when necessary must take independent disciplinary or preventive action for this purpose.

In the author's view, a license to practice medicine is both a privilege and a property right. As a privilege, it is granted by the state with the expectation that licensees will continue to behave in a professionally responsible manner. As valuable private property, a license once granted by the state should be removed or restricted only through due process, when the board has evidence that the licensee's behavior was, or is, not up to professional standards. The courts are available to ensure due process and the protection of licensees' rights against arbitrary actions of the board. In a given case, when these two opposing concepts of licensure— privilege and property right—are in direct conflict, boards try to act in ways that protect the public health and safety. This latter concern, after all, is the central reason for the state boards' licensing power. In adjudicating disputed cases, courts usually defer to the boards on issues of health, safety, and professional competence, but they exercise final authority when a case turns on matters of legal rights and due process.

State regulation of medical practitioners is therefore fundamentally different from state regulation of industry and of business executives. Medical practitioners are not in essence commercial vendors, although they earn their livelihood from payments for their services. Neither is medical care in essence a commodity, although it is now being bought and sold in what many refer to as a "market." In a landmark decision in 1975, the Supreme Court decided that the reach of the federal antitrust laws extended to the professions, including law and medicine.[1] By that decision, the Court seemed to be saying, among other things, that the economic aspects of the practice of medicine resembled business closely enough to warrant antitrust regulation. It seems obvious to the author that the medical care delivery system should not, and cannot, be regulated as if it were simply a commercial market.[2] Sick, frightened, and worried patients are not "consumers" in the ordinary sense of the word, and the relation between them and their doctors is not like that between customers and business people or vendors. Unlike vendors, physicians are expected to take responsibility for counseling and caring for their patients. For their part, patients depend on the expert knowledge, skills, and compassion of their physicians. This trusting relationship has no parallel in the world of business. State boards, in meeting their public responsibility to regulate practitioners, should intrude as little as possible into that relationship, but they should hold physicians accountable for how they behave toward patients. Boards take their own disciplinary action when necessary, although they also rely heavily on the self-monitoring behavior of the profession, and occasionally on the courts. State agencies responsible for regulating commerce cannot, and do not, rely at all on businesses to monitor themselves, nor do they expect businesses to act as fiduciaries and counselors for the customer.

The growth of managed care and the increasing corporatization of medical services do not change the need for state regulation of doctors, nor lessen the responsibility of professional organizations for peer review and quality assurance. Many proponents of the new corporate medicine would argue that oversight of practitioners by business managers will, to a significant degree, replace oversight by the state and the profession itself. They claim that practice guidelines, reporting of outcomes, and the use of an increasing number of putative measures of "quality" will protect patients against substandard care and identify incompetent practitioners, as will the more systematic attention by healthcare companies to selection and certification of doctors. Indeed, in their ads many HMO companies try to reassure the public about the excellent personal care they provide, as if the organization itself were responsible for the quality of professional medical services. However, this emphasis on the reliability of the corporate brand overlooks some essential facts. Although HMO business managers can influence the behavior of their physicians through their control of financial incentives, they have no standing in the clinical management of patients. They usually have no medical competence, and even if they happen to be MDs, they have no direct professional responsibility for individual patients and often are not even licensed to practice medicine in the states where the care is being given. Furthermore, HMO business managers are primarily accountable to their corporate bosses, who serve the private financial interests of the company. Concern for the public interest and the protection of patients does not receive the highest priority as it does in a public licensing authority.

Most states limit the practice of medicine to "natural persons" who are licensed physicians, thereby excluding other legal entities such as corporations. Some states even have laws explicitly prohibiting the "corporate practice of medicine." Legal niceties aside, sick patients need to be taken care of by "natural persons" who are professional caregivers, such as physicians and nurses. However reassuring the company brand name may be, and whatever the reputation of the corporation, no organization can substitute for a personal physician in taking direct responsibility for medical care. This is not to deny that healthcare organizations such as hospitals and HMOs are important elements in the medical care system. They certainly are, and the quality and efficiency with which they function as organizations may greatly affect the care patients receive. But there is no escaping the fact that physicians are the key professionals involved in caring for the sick in our society. State law allows other licensed healthcare professionals to assume limited responsibilities, but only physicians can take full responsibility for the diagnosis and treatment of patients.

Organizations cannot replace physicians in the care of the sick, but organizations in which physicians work can help their doctors regulate the quality of medical care. As a condition of licensure, hospitals are expected to have formal quality assurance procedures in place. Credentialing, peer review of physician behavior, and tracking of outcomes and complications are examples of the way well-run hospitals help physicians organize and maintain effective professional self-regulation. In some states, Massachusetts for example, medical licensing boards work with hospitals to promote quality assurance, and in most states, hospitals are required to report to the state board disciplinary actions taken by their medical staff. Group practices and staff-model and group-model HMOs promote many kinds of formal, and informal, educational and monitoring functions that contribute to professional self-regulation. Even a few of the better independent practice association–type HMOs do something similar for the office-based physicians in their network. In all these examples, however, the organization facilitates and oversees professional peer review and quality improvement by physicians. It cannot replace the physicians' self-regulating function, just as it cannot substitute for the direct care-giving responsibility of the doctors.

What about the claim that continuous monitoring and objective measurement of quality by healthcare organizations can play a major new role in protecting patients, thereby reducing the need for other forms of regulation? This is a laudable theoretical goal, but unattainable now and for the foreseeable future. Quality measurement is an infant science and is not likely to mature for a long time. Some reliable measures of preventive and routine care have been developed and there are methods for assessing outcomes for a few defined procedures and treatments. But there are very few tools for the objective measurement of quality of care when patients are severely ill, that is, when medical professional services are most urgently needed and when competence and integrity count the most. Corporate business management, with its focus on profits and economic efficiency, is no substitute for the public and private professional mechanisms on which society currently relies on to regulate and oversee the quality of medical practitioners and the work they do.

The consumer movement is said to offer another approach to reducing the need for state regulation of medical practice. In theory, adequately informed patients should be able to make better judgments about the quality of their care and the competence of their physicians than uninformed patients can. The author agrees with this idea and favors giving patients, whenever possible, as much information as they want. The fact remains, however, that there is a substantial and irreducible asymmetry between what most patients can understand about their health problems and what their physician knows. Anybody who is ever very sick or seriously injured quickly learns the importance of being able to depend on the counsel and help of a trusted physician. In any case, even well-informed patients need to depend on the state board for certifying the competence of their physicians and need to rely on the fact that bad and dangerous doctors will be removed from practice. Only the most zealous of libertarians would argue that *anyone*, regardless of professional education, licensure, and certification, ought to be allowed to practice medicine. Few would wish to contemplate the horrendous consequences of eliminating licensure requirements, on the theory that they limit competition by restricting entry into a free market.

This brings the discussion to the subject of applying antitrust law to the private self-regulation of the medical profession. As noted in Chapter 7, state regulation has rarely been challenged on antitrust grounds, but private self-regulation (i.e., certification, credentialing, and peer review by professional organizations) has been the subject of much antitrust litigation. Courts have often been unmoved by the argument that private regulation by the profession should be exempted from antitrust laws because the purpose of that regulation is to protect the public from substandard practitioners. The courts are not nearly as comfortable with technical issues of professional quality and the protection of public health as they are with legal matters like antitrust. Therefore, they concentrate on their legal agenda, leaving the public health issues to be resolved by the other branches of government. In any event, professional peer review in hospitals and physicians' organizations has frequently been intimidated by the prospect of being challenged in the courts. Many a physician has chosen not to be a whistle-blower against an incompetent colleague for fear of having to defend himself against antitrust legal action brought by the accused. National accrediting bodies have not yet faced serious antitrust challenge, but this remains a possibility. The basic view of the antitrust enforcing agencies and the courts seems to be that medicine is a market like any other, and the preservation of competition should take precedence over all other considerations. In accord with this view, some antitrust advocates have even suggested the possibility of promoting competition among accrediting agencies as a way of resolving the tension between the market and private regulation. In the author's opinion, such proposals are specious because the premises upon which they are based are false. As argued above, medical practice is not primarily a business, and the medical care system is not primarily a market. Current trends toward its commercialization notwithstanding, the ineluctable fact remains that healthcare serves different purposes than commerce, and medical practitioners are not only, or even primarily, tradespeople. That is why the regulation of medical practice must be different from the regulation of ordinary trade, and why the concepts of market competition cannot be directly applied to medicine.

How Do the Boards Work? The Impressions of a Physician Member

State boards vary in their procedures and their effectiveness, so it is difficult to make general statements that apply with equal force to all. The author's personal experience is limited to membership on the Board of Registration in Medicine of the Commonwealth of Massachusetts, but the following comments also draw on general information obtained from the annual reports of the Federation of State Medical Boards and from other published materials.

The state boards are in transition. Decades ago, most of their activity was confined to licensing and occasional disciplinary responses to egregious breaches of professional conduct. Twelve years ago the author wrote an editorial in the *New England Journal of Medicine* calling attention to the extraordinary variation among state boards in the annual frequency of their disciplinary actions.[3] According to the Federation of State Medical Boards, the number of disciplinary actions in 1982 ranged from 0 to 7.4 per thousand licensed physicians. Seventeen states reported 3.0 or more actions per thousand that year, but fifteen states reported 1.0 or fewer. Among the largest states, those with 10,000 or more licensed physicians, Florida had the highest rate (7.4 per thousand) and Pennsylvania the lowest (0.5 per thousand). Those statistics have gradually changed, but there is still great variation among states. According to a 1995 report from the FSMB[4] there were no states taking no disciplinary actions that year, and the number varied from 0.6 to 15.4 per thousand, with a median of 5.2

actions. Some of this variation is probably due to technical differences in definitions and procedures among the states, but state boards undoubtedly continue to oversee their licensees with varying diligence and effectiveness, because it is hard to imagine that physicians differ as much in quality among the various states as the differences in discipline rates might otherwise suggest. There is no way to know what disciplinary rate would be "appropriate," but the author's experience would suggest the median rate ought to be substantially higher than is now being reported, and the variation among states should be less. The most likely explanation for this variation is that state boards labor under several handicaps that affect their functioning to varying degrees.

Inadequate Resources

Operating budgets are low, thereby limiting the number and quality of a board's legal and administrative staff. Data management capacity is often woefully inadequate. Board members are usually paid only token stipends, so for practical purposes they are being asked to serve pro bono. For most board members, this means they can spare relatively little time for their board duties and must rely heavily on the staff. This is no problem for much of the board's routine work, but investigation and adjudication of complicated cases and development of board regulations and public policies require a level of sustained effort that most board members are unable to give. Excessive demands on the time of underpaid board members cause rapid turnover in membership, which also impairs a board's efficiency. Modest increases in the average size of the board might help, but would not entirely solve the problem. The use of pro bono consultants and outside review panels, while of great help in some respects, would not solve the problem either. The net result of inadequate resources, for many boards, is delayed attention to pending cases, lapses in routine functions, and inability to develop and pursue new policies. In some states there are delays of up to several years in the resolution of cases.

Board Appointments

The appointment process for new members of the board is often heavily political, and there is not enough effort to obtain the best people available. Good staff are essential for the effective work of all boards, of course, but good, conscientious board members are no less critical. Many excellent physicians and first-rate public members serve on boards throughout the country, but the quality of board membership is unfortunately not uniform and many available and highly qualified people are never asked to serve. What is needed in most states is a more systematic process for selecting and appointing new members that is essentially free of politics and cronyism. Given the realities of most state governments, this is probably an unattainable goal.

Perceptions of Boards

There is an unfortunate suspicion of the boards by physicians, hospital medical staffs, and many state medical organizations. Most physicians feel threatened by the state boards and want to have nothing to do with them. They are also reluctant to cooperate in filing reports about colleagues. Ideally, organized medicine and medical care institutions should be working together with state boards to protect the public safety and the good name of the profession, but that is not often the case. It is unrealistic to expect that physicians would welcome regulation and discipline by state boards, although most of them recognize that the boards are doing what must be done, and what the profession cannot do by itself. However, there is certainly much room for improvement in existing relations. This would undoubtedly be facilitated if board members were better known and more respected by their professional medical colleagues. Relations would also be improved if boards were seen not only as disciplinary agencies, but as agencies committed to rehabilitation and remediation of impaired and substandard physicians. At present the relationship between the boards and the medical profession is more adversarial than it ought to be. The effectiveness with which each board does its job therefore depends in part upon how aggressively its members and staff are willing to pursue their regulatory responsibilities, despite the lack of cooperation—or even the resistance—of medical professionals and their organizations.

Difficult Cases

Drug-dependent or psychiatrically impaired physicians constitute the major share of the cases now coming before the boards, but dealing with them is difficult, discouraging, and tedious. Management of such cases is often undertaken by special organizations established by state medical societies with the cooperation and oversight of the boards. In Massachusetts the state medical society has established a nonprofit corporation called Physician's Health Service, which puts voluntarily referred physicians into treatment and monitoring programs. This is handled confidentially, unless a disciplinary action has been taken, which then, as a matter of law, must be on the public record. The state board refers many physicians to Physician's Health Service and relies on regular reports from the latter to determine what further disciplinary action need be taken, and whether a previously impaired physician is ready to return to practice. It is a system that works well in Massachusetts and deserves to be more widely adopted.

More Difficult Cases

Substandard or incompetent physicians are a potentially greater problem for state boards than even drug-dependent or psychiatrically impaired physicians, and yet there are no generally accepted procedures for dealing with them. Renewal of medical licensure in most states requires that applicants complete a certain minimum number of hours of CME. Most specialty boards now require recertification examinations at certain pre-scribed intervals. However, CME credits do not guarantee competence, and even board-certified specialists may find themselves in areas of practice for which they are inadequately trained. Among the major advantages of group practice and membership on the medical staff of teaching hospitals are the continuous professional peer oversight and educational experience such appointments provide. All well-run hospitals have peer-review mechanisms that check on the qualifications and privileges of their staff members, and continuously monitor performance. Mishaps are reviewed, and serious ones due to professional incompetence may come to a board's attention for disciplinary action. Much of the variation in rates of disciplinary action among states may be due to variations in the effectiveness of their systems for the identification of seriously incompetent practitioners. In the absence of serious mishaps to patients, dangerously substandard physicians may escape attention for a long time.

Procedural Impediments

Boards are often impeded in their consideration of relatively straightfor-ward medical issues by excessive procedural rules and legal restraints. It is important, of course, to ensure due process and to protect licensees' rights against arbitrary disciplinary actions. However, these legitimate concerns may often be carried too far. As a result, boards are often frustrated in their attempts to investigate cases and reach decisions expeditiously. This problem exists to a varying degree among the boards, and it undoubtedly accounts for some of the variations in numbers of completed disciplinary actions. In Massachusetts, one of the most frus-trating examples of excessive legal restraint is a court ruling that allows hospitals to withhold many essential details in a case being investigated by the board, on the grounds that these details are part of the "peer review" proceedings of the medical staff and, as such, are protected from disclosure.[5] In principle, there is some rationale to this ruling, but in practice it is often employed to keep the board from learning facts necessary for it to do its job of protecting the public interest. Physicians and hospitals are understandably worried about the public disclosure that results when the board takes disciplinary action, and they fear that any involvement with the board will bring damaging publicity. Despite the fact that earlier stages of an investigation are held in confidence, there is much concern about this. Some hospitals cooperate only reluctantly with the board, and only under tight protective restraints by their lawyers.

Considering all the handicaps under which they labor, the state boards have done well to perform as they do. They should do even better, but they will have to solve some of the problems enumerated above, and they will have to respond effectively to the rapidly changing shape of the U.S. healthcare system.

The Future of Regulation

As already noted, state boards are in transition. They are changing, and will continue to change, not only because they are trying to become more effective at what they are already doing, but also because they are confronting a rapidly evolving medical care system.

An increasing fraction of medical care is being provided outside of hospitals. HMOs and other managed care systems are largely based on ambulatory services. Much of the treatment previously given in hospitals is now provided in outpatient facilities. As the use of hospitals is reduced, so too are the regulatory functions they formerly provided through peer review and medical staff oversight. If these functions are to be sustained, they will have to be provided by the ambulatory care facilities, by the HMOs and the other kinds of integrated medical care delivery systems that are replacing the hospitals. In the future, boards will have to count on these new systems to monitor physician behavior and report critical incidents. However, most state boards do not yet have the kinds of relations with these ambulatory systems that they have developed with hospitals. New statutory authority, as well as new procedures and relationships will have to be established for this purpose. Otherwise, large parts of medical practice will escape peer review and thereby avoid oversight by the boards.

The rapid pace of technological and scientific advances in medicine will also put new demands on state boards. Physicians who have completed their training more than a few years ago are finding it more difficult to stay current in their knowledge and skills. As noted above, substandard competence is becoming an ever-increasing problem, which now poses a greater threat to the public health and safety than drug-dependent and psychiatrically impaired physicians. Boards will soon need to confront this problem, and will need to develop procedures to identify substandard practitioners. Some of these practitioners will need discipline, but most will need help in improving their skills. Such physicians should have the opportunity voluntarily to refer themselves (or accept referral) to specially designed remediation programs, at their own expense, and without the stigma of a formal disciplinary action. Many complaints now coming to the Massachusetts board—and, most likely, to most other boards—are concerned with physicians in this category. Boards should be able to make mandatory referrals to such programs when necessary, as an alternative to formal discipline or outright dismissal of the case. The Massachusetts Medical Society and state board are now considering such a program. If it proves effective and affordable, it will deserve wide adoption.

State boards are working together more closely than ever before, but they will have to cooperate even more in the future. The FSMB has done much to bring the boards into closer contact with one another, but they still remain legally independent entities under the jurisdiction of separate sovereign states. Despite the many avenues of cooperation and communication opened up by the FSMB, there is still much unnecessary duplication and overlap of function among the boards. Telemedicine is a case in point. Technological advances in this field now make it possible for a patient in one state to receive a diagnostic evaluation by a physician living in, and licensed by, another state. In principle, such a physician is "practicing medicine without a license" in the state where the patient resides. Unless the benefits of telemedicine are to be seriously restricted, state boards will have to agree on some uniform modifications in their licensing regulations to permit physicians to diagnose across state boundaries. The FSMB is actively working on this problem. This is only one instance among many in which the public interest would be better served by a future state board system that is less decentralized and better integrated on a national level.

In conclusion, the present regulation of the medical profession by state boards leaves much to be desired. However, most existing problems could be solved by more efficient administration, and better support, of the boards, and by more cooperation from the profession. Although the present reality is far from ideal, some of the recent developments outlined above offer hope of substantial improvement in the near future. In any case, it seems clear that the medical profession will not thrive unless it accepts the need for increased public accountability—and that will inevitably require more regulation.

Notes

1. *Goldfarb v. Virginia State Bar*, 421 U.S. 773 (1975).

2. A. S. Relman. 1985. "Antitrust Law and the Physician Entrepreneur." *New England Journal of Medicine* 313 (14): 884.

3. A. S. Relman. 1985. "Professional Regulation and the State Medical Boards." *New England Journal of Medicine* 312 (12): 784.

4. Federation of State Medical Boards of the United States, Inc. "Summary of 1995 Board Actions." April 2, 1996.

5. *Beth Israel Hospital Association v. Board of Registration in Medicine*, 401 Mass. 172 (1987).

INDEX

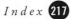

CONTRIBUTORS

Timothy Stoltzfus Jost, J.D., the editor and a chapter author, is the Newton Baker, Baker and Hostetler Professor of Law at The Ohio State University. He is also a professor of Health Services Management and Policy in The Ohio State University College of Medicine.

    Linda H. Aiken, Ph.D., is Trustee Professor of Nursing, Professor of Sociology, and Director for Health Services and Policy Research at the University of Pennsylvania. She is a member of the Institute of Medicine, a former president of the American Academy of Nursing, and a member of the Physician Payment Review Commission.

    Thomas L. Greaney, J.D., is a Professor of Law at St. Louis University School of Law. Prior to beginning his teaching career, he served for over a decade at the U.S. Department of Justice, where he was the Assistant Chief of the Antitrust Division, supervising health industry matters from 1982 to 1986.

    Joyce M. Greenleaf, M.B.A., is a project leader in the Office of Evaluation and Inspections, Office of Inspector General, Department of Health and Human Services, in Boston.

    Sandra H. Johnson, J.D., is Professor of Law at the Center for Health Law Studies of the St. Louis University School of Law. She holds appointments as Associate Professor of Law and Medicine and Professor of Law in Health Care Administration at the University's Schools of Medicine and Public Health.

    Eleanor Kinney, J.D., M.P.H., is Professor of Law and Director of the Center for Law and Health at Indiana University School of Law–Indianapolis. She is also an adjunct professor of Public and Environmental Affairs at Indiana University.

David Orentlicher, M.D., J.D., is Associate Professor of Law, Indiana University School of Law–Indianapolis, and Adjunct Associate Professor of Medicine, Indiana School of Medicine. He was formerly Director of the Division of Medical Ethics of the American Medical Association.

Arnold S. Relman, M.D., is Professor Emeritus of Medicine and of Social Medicine at the Harvard Medical School and Editor-in-Chief Emeritus of the *New England Journal of Medicine.* He is a fellow of the American Academy of Arts and Sciences, a member of the Institute of Medicine, and a member of the Board of Registration in Medicine of the Commonwealth of Massachusetts.

William M. Sage, M.D., J.D., is an Associate Professor of Law and Adjunct Assistant Professor of Medicine at Columbia University. He headed four working groups of the White House Task Force on Health Care Reform and has been a corporate health law attorney at O'Melveny & Myers in Los Angeles.

Mark R. Yessian, Ph.D., is Regional Inspector General for Evaluation and Inspections in the Department of Health and Human Services. In the past he has been a special assistant in the Office of the Secretary of DHHS, an Assistant Professor of Public Management at Suffolk University, and Director of Policy Analysis for the Oklahoma Department of Human Services.